# Differential Diagnosis Diagrams: Fast Focus Study Guide

JT Thomas, MD

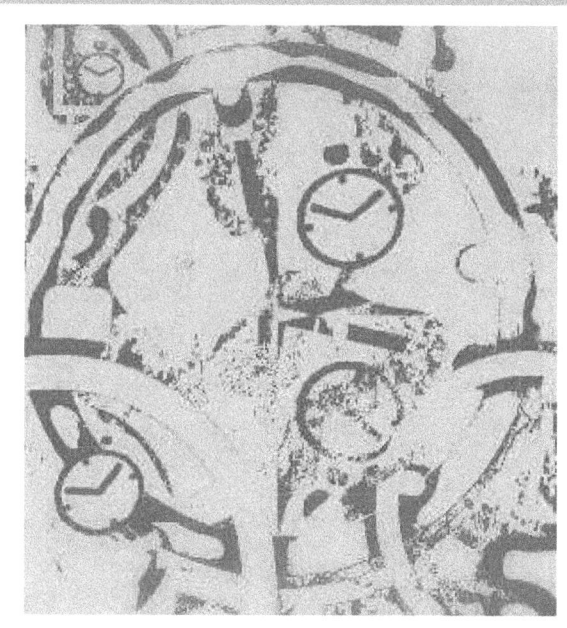

# CONTENTS

- This book is written to help the reader further visualize and determine the differential diagnosis for common medical conditions.

- This book is written in a simple and easy to read format.

- This book simplifies a complicated medical issue so you will remember the important details.

- You will not get caught up in the minutia.

- This Fast Focus Study Guide will provide you with a practical review of the key information you need to know.

- Buy this book now if you want this quick and concise information

Table of Contents:

# Acute Abdomen

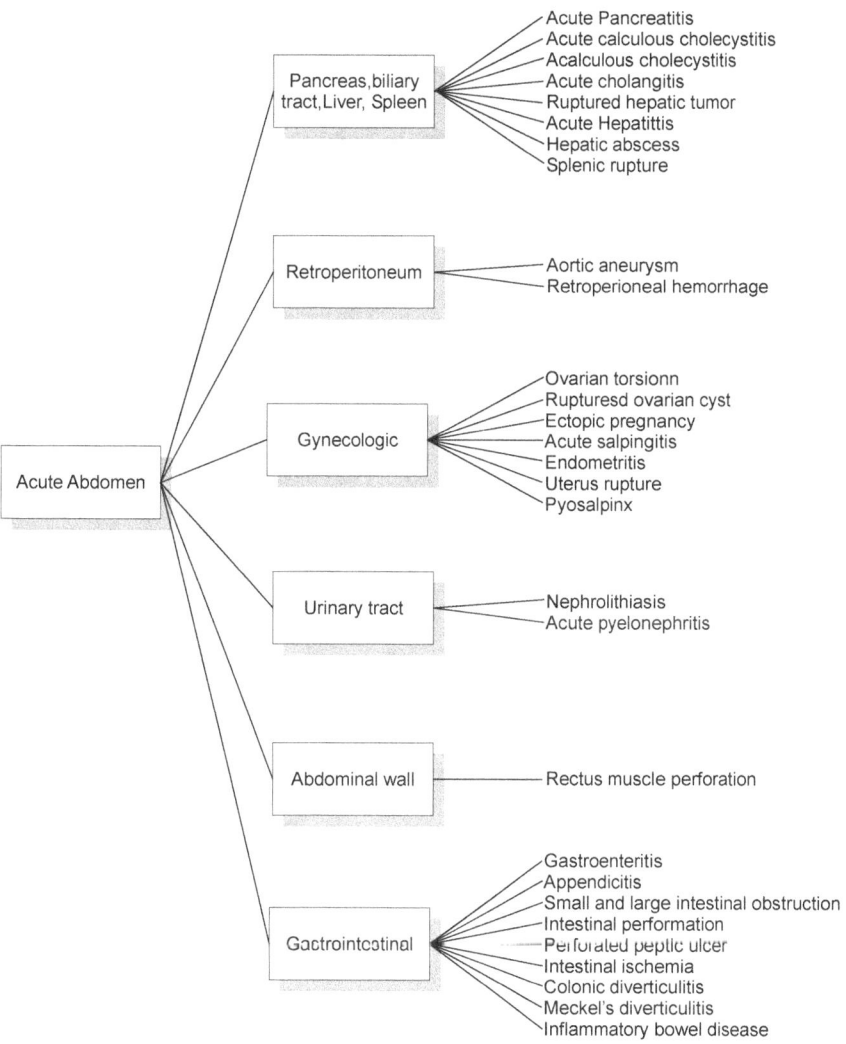

Reference: Martin R, Rossi R. Abdominal emergencies: Has anything changed? The acute abdomen. Surgical Clin North America 1997;77(6):1227.

# Acute Renal Failure

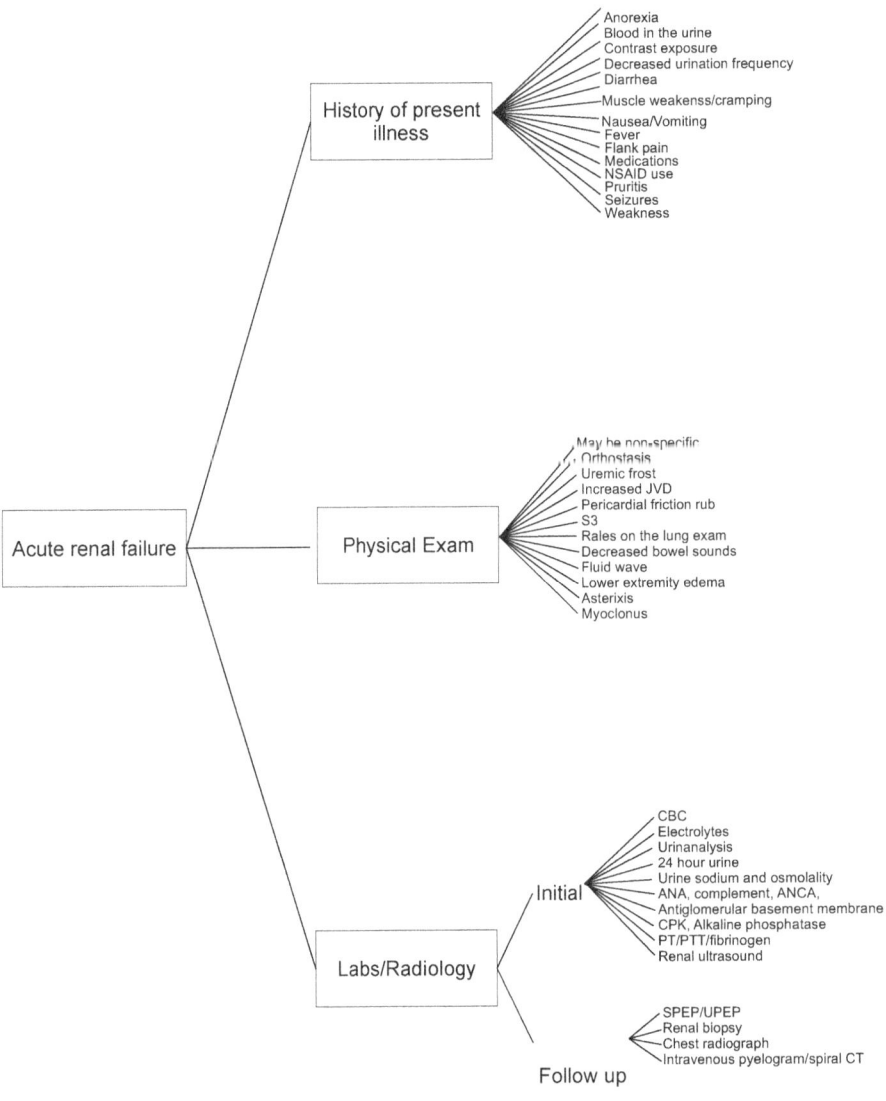

**History of present illness**
- Anorexia
- Blood in the urine
- Contrast exposure
- Decreased urination frequency
- Diarrhea
- Muscle weakenss/cramping
- Nausea/Vomiting
- Fever
- Flank pain
- Medications
- NSAID use
- Pruritis
- Seizures
- Weakness

**Acute renal failure**

**Physical Exam**
- May be non-specific
- Orthostasis
- Uremic frost
- Increased JVD
- Pericardial friction rub
- S3
- Rales on the lung exam
- Decreased bowel sounds
- Fluid wave
- Lower extremity edema
- Asterixis
- Myoclonus

**Labs/Radiology**

Initial
- CBC
- Electrolytes
- Urinanalysis
- 24 hour urine
- Urine sodium and osmolality
- ANA, complement, ANCA,
- Antiglomerular basement membrane
- CPK, Alkaline phosphatase
- PT/PTT/fibrinogen
- Renal ultrasound

- SPEP/UPEP
- Renal biopsy
- Chest radiograph
- Intravenous pyelogram/spiral CT

Follow up

# Primary Adrenocortical Insufficiency

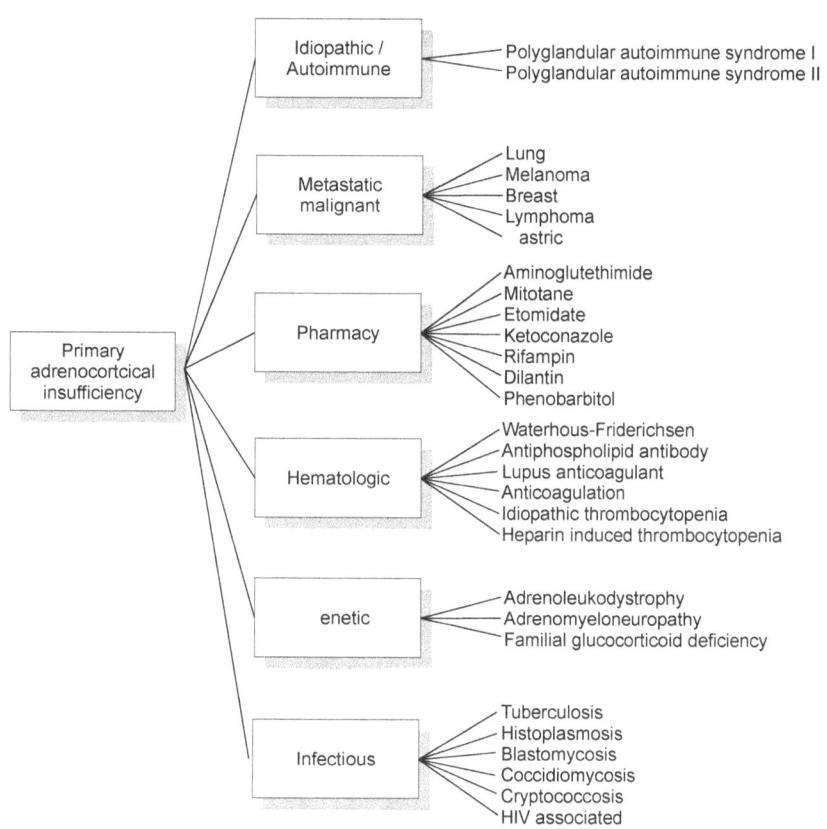

Primary adrenocortcical insufficiency

- Idiopathic / Autoimmune
  - Polyglandular autoimmune syndrome I
  - Polyglandular autoimmune syndrome II
- Metastatic malignant
  - Lung
  - Melanoma
  - Breast
  - Lymphoma
  - astric
- Pharmacy
  - Aminoglutethimide
  - Mitotane
  - Etomidate
  - Ketoconazole
  - Rifampin
  - Dilantin
  - Phenobarbitol
- Hematologic
  - Waterhous-Friderichsen
  - Antiphospholipid antibody
  - Lupus anticoagulant
  - Anticoagulation
  - Idiopathic thrombocytopenia
  - Heparin induced thrombocytopenia
- enetic
  - Adrenoleukodystrophy
  - Adrenomyeloneuropathy
  - Familial glucocorticoid deficiency
- Infectious
  - Tuberculosis
  - Histoplasmosis
  - Blastomycosis
  - Coccidiomycosis
  - Cryptococcosis
  - HIV associated

Reference  Werbel S, Ober P Acute adrenal insufficiency  Endocrinology and metabolism clinics of North America 22  3  3-32

# Amenorrhea

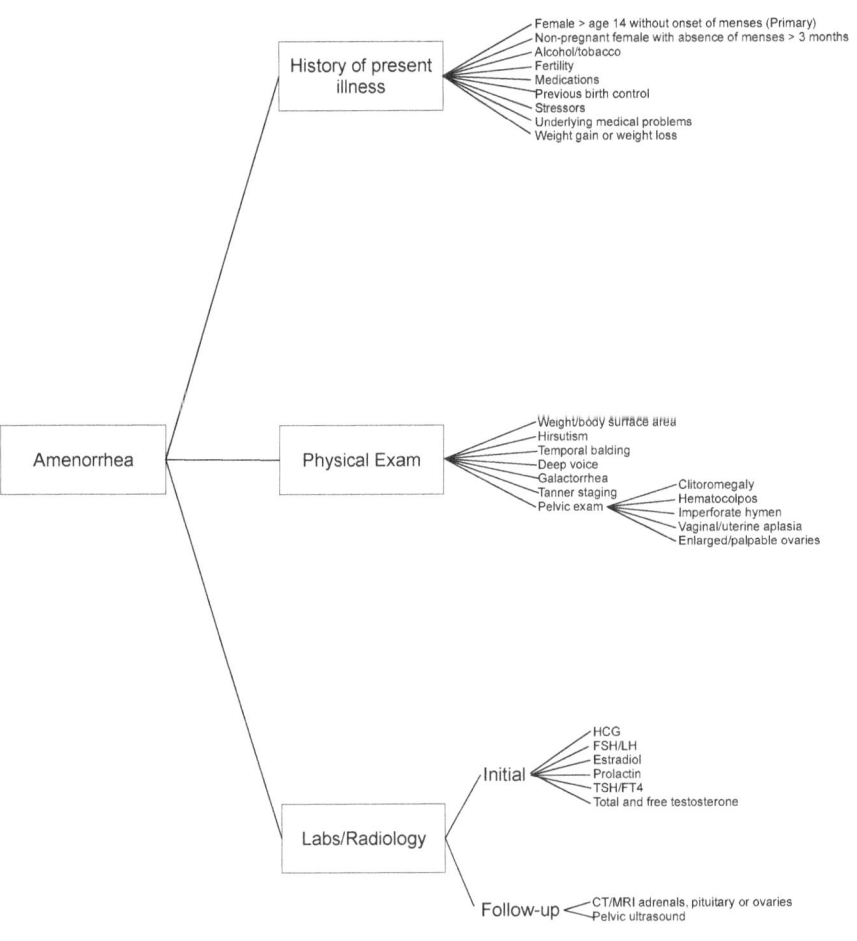

**Amenorrhea**

**History of present illness**
- Female > age 14 without onset of menses (Primary)
- Non-pregnant female with absence of menses > 3 months
- Alcohol/tobacco
- Fertility
- Medications
- Previous birth control
- Stressors
- Underlying medical problems
- Weight gain or weight loss

**Physical Exam**
- Weight/body surface area
- Hirsutism
- Temporal balding
- Deep voice
- Galactorrhea
- Tanner staging
- Pelvic exam
  - Clitoromegaly
  - Hematocolpos
  - Imperforate hymen
  - Vaginal/uterine aplasia
  - Enlarged/palpable ovaries

**Labs/Radiology**
- Initial
  - HCG
  - FSH/LH
  - Estradiol
  - Prolactin
  - TSH/FT4
  - Total and free testosterone
- Follow-up
  - CT/MRI adrenals, pituitary or ovaries
  - Pelvic ultrasound

# Hemolytic Anemia

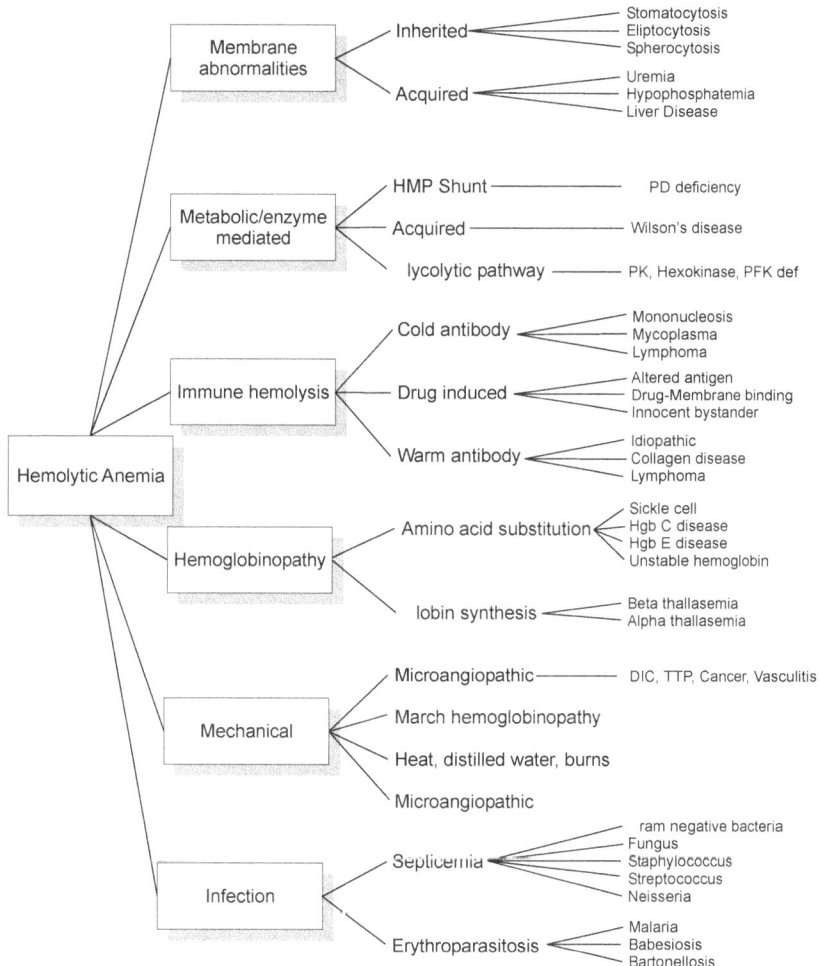

Reference  Smith L  Autoimmune hemolytic anemias  characteristics and classification  Clin Lab Sci     2 2     -4

# Anemia

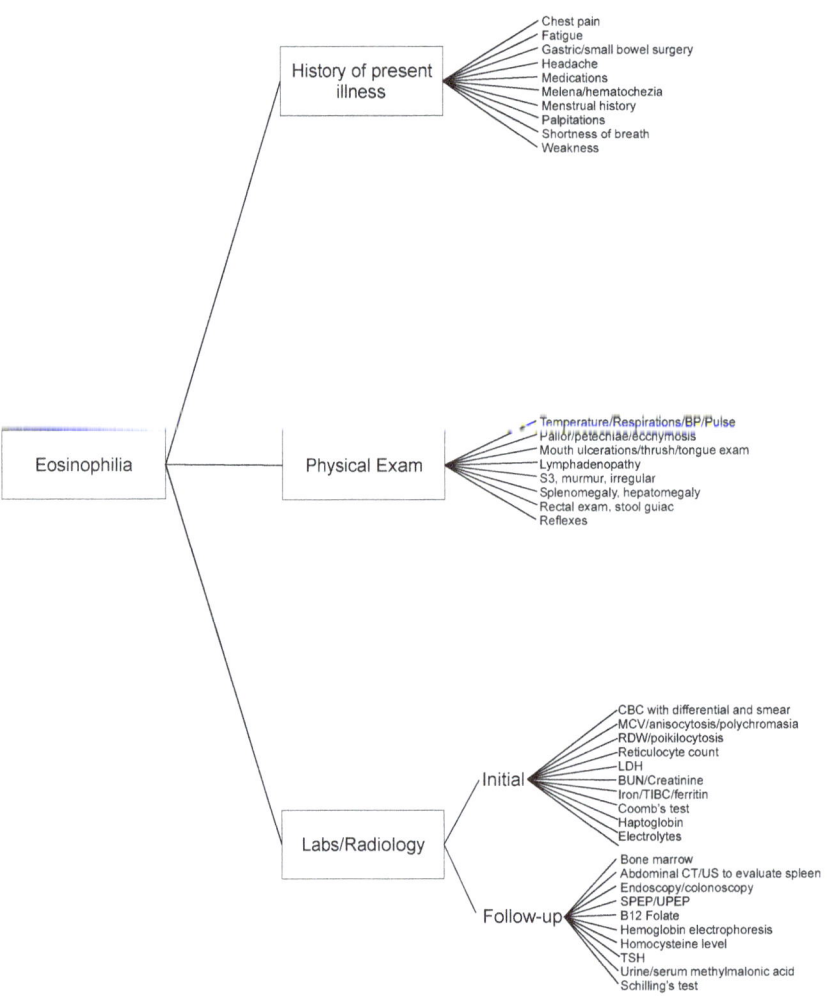

**History of present illness**
- Chest pain
- Fatigue
- Gastric/small bowel surgery
- Headache
- Medications
- Melena/hematochezia
- Menstrual history
- Palpitations
- Shortness of breath
- Weakness

**Eosinophilia**

**Physical Exam**
- Temperature/Respirations/BP/Pulse
- Pallor/petechiae/ecchymosis
- Mouth ulcerations/thrush/tongue exam
- Lymphadenopathy
- S3, murmur, irregular
- Splenomegaly, hepatomegaly
- Rectal exam, stool guiac
- Reflexes

**Labs/Radiology**

*Initial*
- CBC with differential and smear
- MCV/anisocytosis/polychromasia
- RDW/poikilocytosis
- Reticulocyte count
- LDH
- BUN/Creatinine
- Iron/TIBC/ferritin
- Coomb's test
- Haptoglobin
- Electrolytes

*Follow-up*
- Bone marrow
- Abdominal CT/US to evaluate spleen
- Endoscopy/colonoscopy
- SPEP/UPEP
- B12 Folate
- Hemoglobin electrophoresis
- Homocysteine level
- TSH
- Urine/serum methylmalonic acid
- Schilling's test

# Anion Gap Acidosis

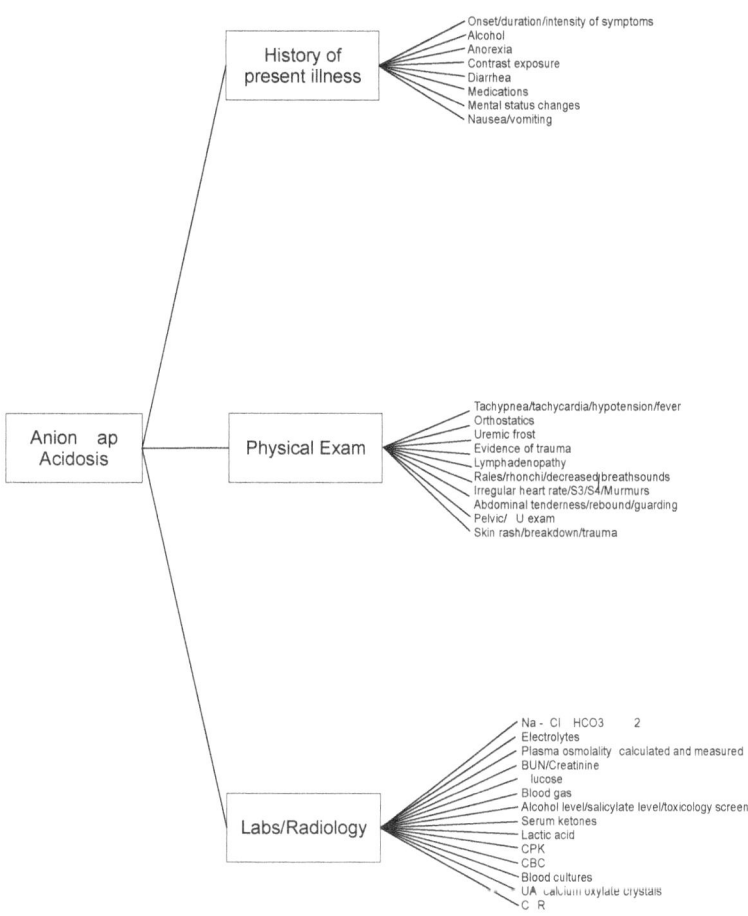

**History of present illness**
- Onset/duration/intensity of symptoms
- Alcohol
- Anorexia
- Contrast exposure
- Diarrhea
- Medications
- Mental status changes
- Nausea/vomiting

**Physical Exam**
- Tachypnea/tachycardia/hypotension/fever
- Orthostatics
- Uremic frost
- Evidence of trauma
- Lymphadenopathy
- Rales/rhonchi/decreased breathsounds
- Irregular heart rate/S3/S4/Murmurs
- Abdominal tenderness/rebound/guarding
- Pelvic/GU exam
- Skin rash/breakdown/trauma

**Labs/Radiology**
- Na - Cl  HCO3       2
- Electrolytes
- Plasma osmolality  calculated and measured
- BUN/Creatinine
- Glucose
- Blood gas
- Alcohol level/salicylate level/toxicology screen
- Serum ketones
- Lactic acid
- CPK
- CBC
- Blood cultures
- UA  calcium oxylate crystals
- C R

# Arrhythmias

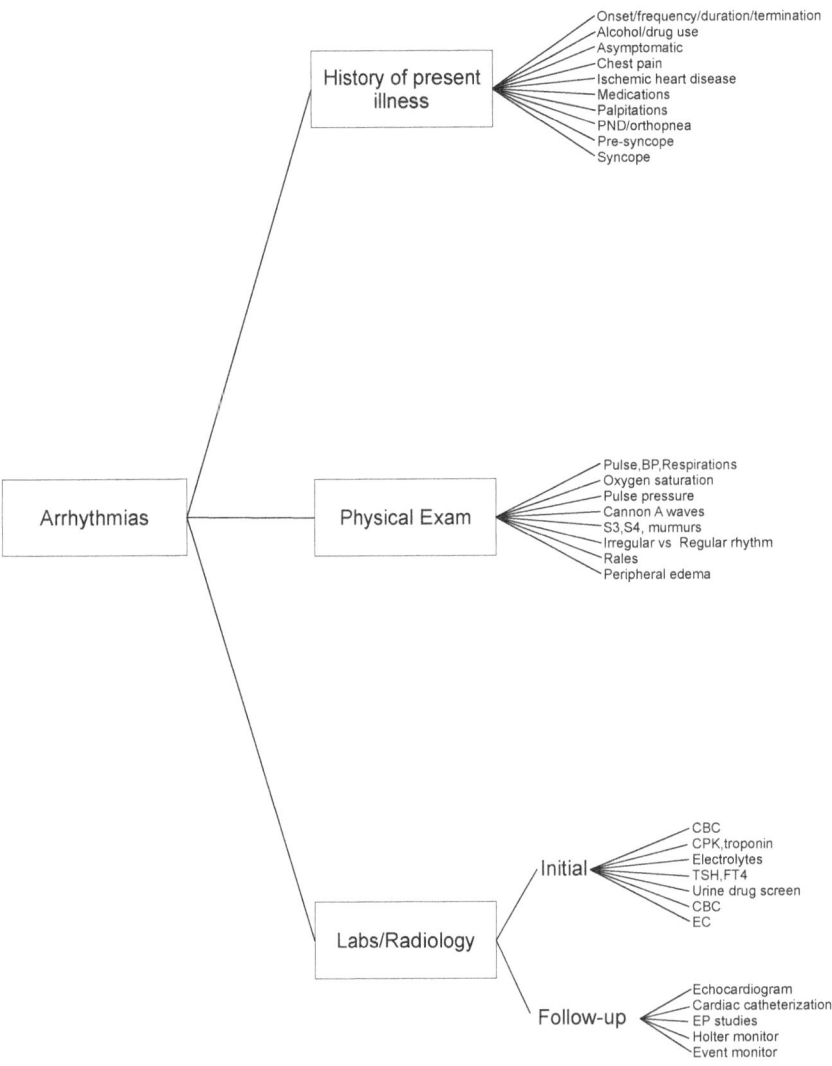

History of present illness
- Onset/frequency/duration/termination
- Alcohol/drug use
- Asymptomatic
- Chest pain
- Ischemic heart disease
- Medications
- Palpitations
- PND/orthopnea
- Pre-syncope
- Syncope

Physical Exam
- Pulse,BP,Respirations
- Oxygen saturation
- Pulse pressure
- Cannon A waves
- S3,S4, murmurs
- Irregular vs Regular rhythm
- Rales
- Peripheral edema

Labs/Radiology

Initial
- CBC
- CPK,troponin
- Electrolytes
- TSH,FT4
- Urine drug screen
- CBC
- EC

Follow-up
- Echocardiogram
- Cardiac catheterization
- EP studies
- Holter monitor
- Event monitor

# Arrhythmias

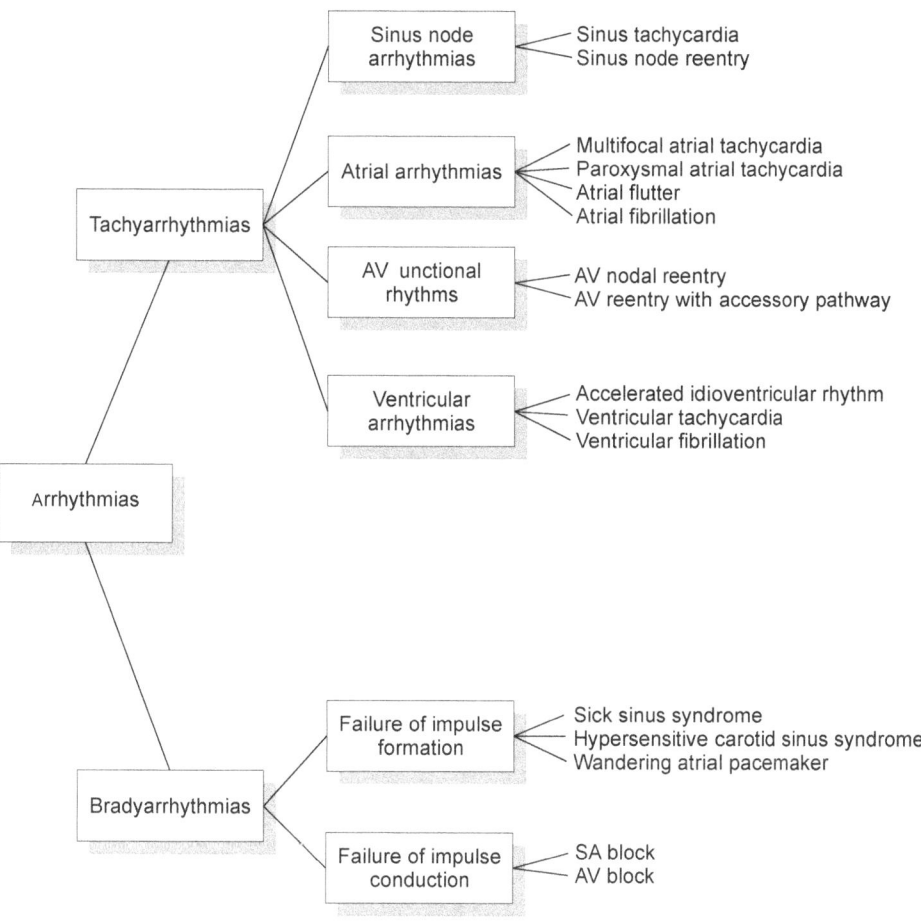

Sinus node arrhythmias
- Sinus tachycardia
- Sinus node reentry

Atrial arrhythmias
- Multifocal atrial tachycardia
- Paroxysmal atrial tachycardia
- Atrial flutter
- Atrial fibrillation

AV unctional rhythms
- AV nodal reentry
- AV reentry with accessory pathway

Ventricular arrhythmias
- Accelerated idioventricular rhythm
- Ventricular tachycardia
- Ventricular fibrillation

Tachyarrhythmias

Arrhythmias

Bradyarrhythmias

Failure of impulse formation
- Sick sinus syndrome
- Hypersensitive carotid sinus syndrome
- Wandering atrial pacemaker

Failure of impulse conduction
- SA block
- AV block

Reference  Janiera L  Wide-complex tachycardias  The importance of identifying the mechanism  Postgrad Med      3 2  -  , 2  - 2
Karas B,   rubb B  Reentrant tachycardias  A look at where treatment stands today  Postgrad Med      2   4-  , 3-  ,

# Ascites

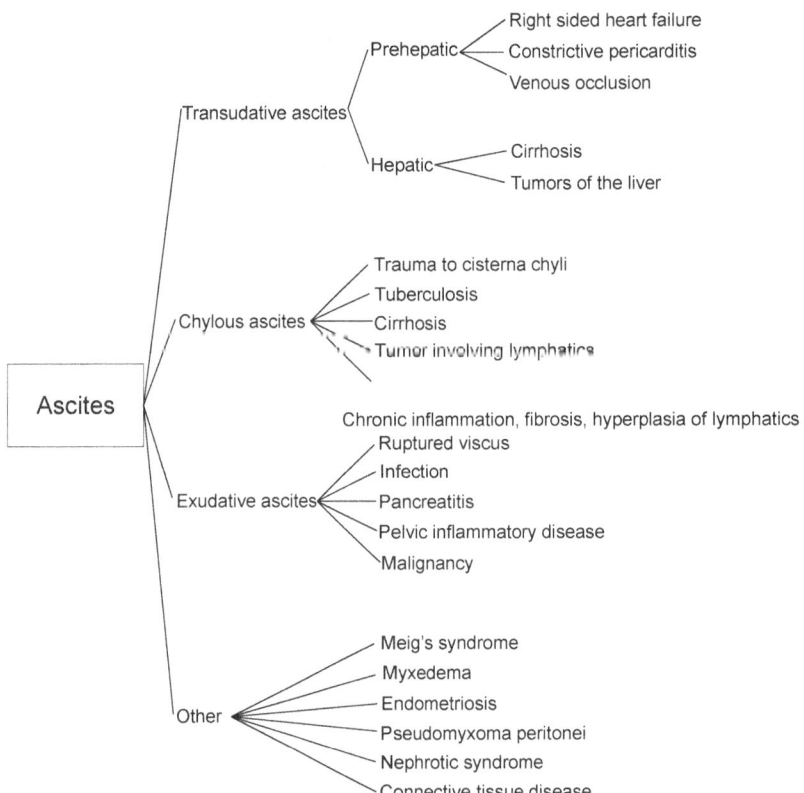

Ascites
- Transudative ascites
  - Prehepatic
    - Right sided heart failure
    - Constrictive pericarditis
    - Venous occlusion
  - Hepatic
    - Cirrhosis
    - Tumors of the liver
- Chylous ascites
  - Trauma to cisterna chyli
  - Tuberculosis
  - Cirrhosis
  - Tumor involving lymphatics
  - Chronic inflammation, fibrosis, hyperplasia of lymphatics
- Exudative ascites
  - Ruptured viscus
  - Infection
  - Pancreatitis
  - Pelvic inflammatory disease
  - Malignancy
- Other
  - Meig's syndrome
  - Myxedema
  - Endometriosis
  - Pseudomyxoma peritonei
  - Nephrotic syndrome
  - Connective tissue disease

Reference: Habeeb K, Herrera J. Management of ascited. Paracentesis as a guide. Postgrad Med 1997;101(1):191-2,195-2001.

# Ascites

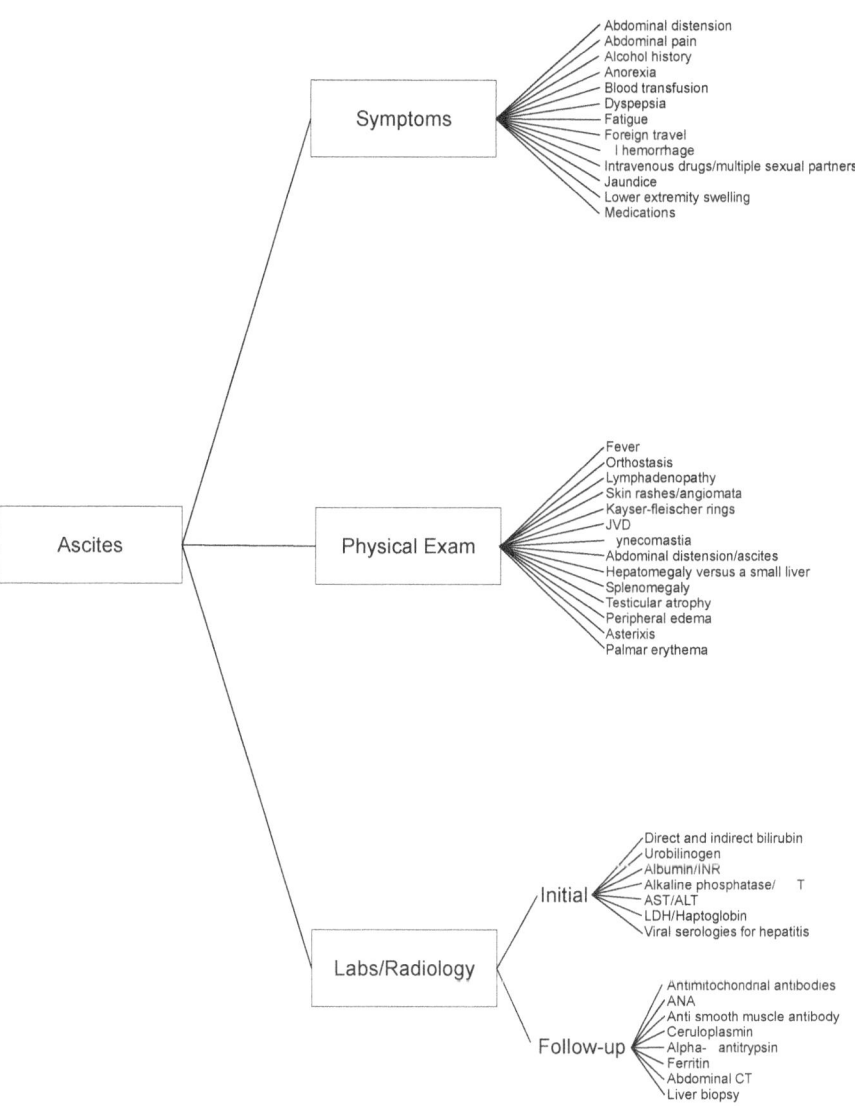

Symptoms
- Abdominal distension
- Abdominal pain
- Alcohol history
- Anorexia
- Blood transfusion
- Dyspepsia
- Fatigue
- Foreign travel
- l hemorrhage
- Intravenous drugs/multiple sexual partners
- Jaundice
- Lower extremity swelling
- Medications

Physical Exam
- Fever
- Orthostasis
- Lymphadenopathy
- Skin rashes/angiomata
- Kayser-fleischer rings
- JVD
- ynecomastia
- Abdominal distension/ascites
- Hepatomegaly versus a small liver
- Splenomegaly
- Testicular atrophy
- Peripheral edema
- Asterixis
- Palmar erythema

Labs/Radiology

Initial
- Direct and indirect bilirubin
- Urobilinogen
- Albumin/INR
- Alkaline phosphatase/    T
- AST/ALT
- LDH/Haptoglobin
- Viral serologies for hepatitis

Follow-up
- Antimitochondnal antibodies
- ANA
- Anti smooth muscle antibody
- Ceruloplasmin
- Alpha-  antitrypsin
- Ferritin
- Abdominal CT
- Liver biopsy

# Atrial Fibrillation

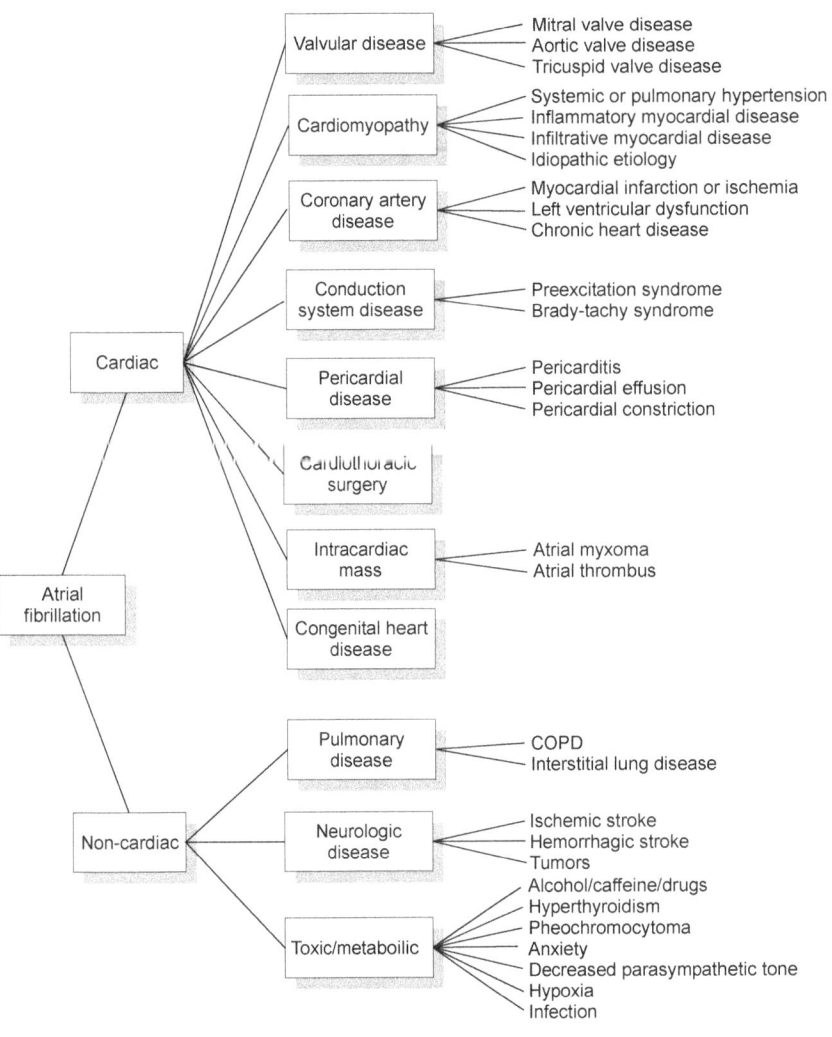

Valvular disease
— Mitral valve disease
— Aortic valve disease
— Tricuspid valve disease

Cardiomyopathy
— Systemic or pulmonary hypertension
— Inflammatory myocardial disease
— Infiltrative myocardial disease
— Idiopathic etiology

Coronary artery disease
— Myocardial infarction or ischemia
— Left ventricular dysfunction
— Chronic heart disease

Conduction system disease
— Preexcitation syndrome
— Brady-tachy syndrome

Pericardial disease
— Pericarditis
— Pericardial effusion
— Pericardial constriction

Cardiothoracic surgery

Intracardiac mass
— Atrial myxoma
— Atrial thrombus

Congenital heart disease

Pulmonary disease
— COPD
— Interstitial lung disease

Neurologic disease
— Ischemic stroke
— Hemorrhagic stroke
— Tumors

Toxic/metaboilic
— Alcohol/caffeine/drugs
— Hyperthyroidism
— Pheochromocytoma
— Anxiety
— Decreased parasympathetic tone
— Hypoxia
— Infection

Cardiac

Atrial fibrillation

Non-cardiac

Reference  Olshansky B, Sulo R  A practical approach to atrial fibrillation  Hospital Practice     May    -

# Atrial Fibrillation

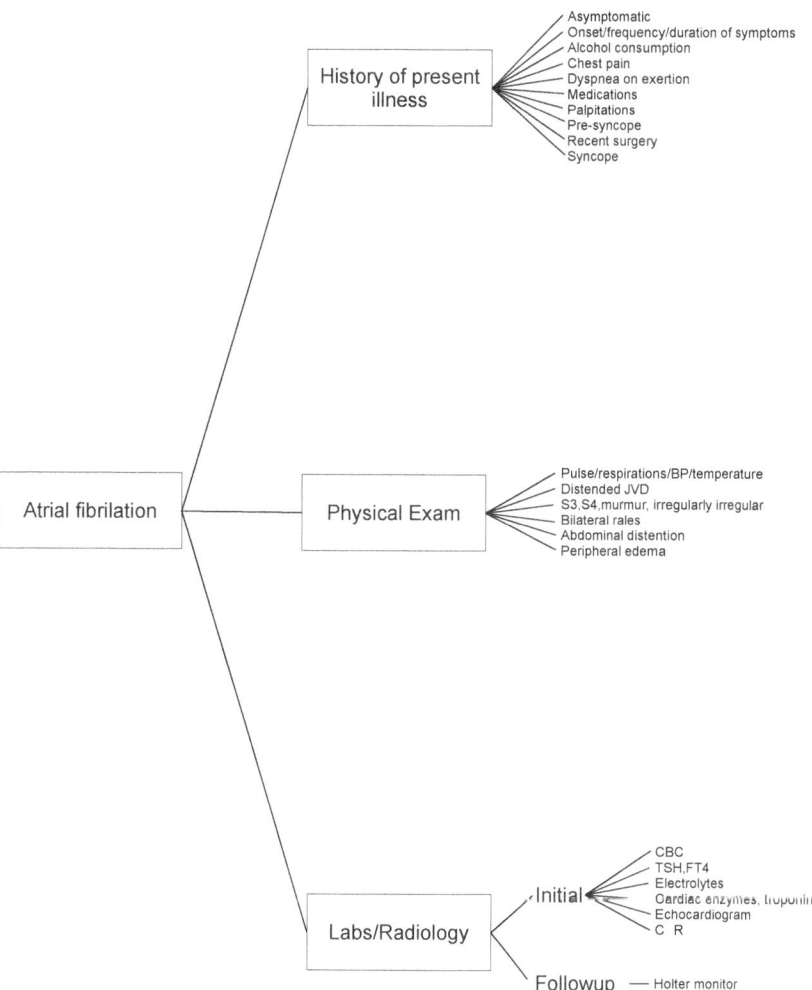

Atrial fibrilation

History of present illness
- Asymptomatic
- Onset/frequency/duration of symptoms
- Alcohol consumption
- Chest pain
- Dyspnea on exertion
- Medications
- Palpitations
- Pre-syncope
- Recent surgery
- Syncope

Physical Exam
- Pulse/respirations/BP/temperature
- Distended JVD
- S3,S4,murmur, irregularly irregular
- Bilateral rales
- Abdominal distention
- Peripheral edema

Labs/Radiology

Initial
- CBC
- TSH,FT4
- Electrolytes
- Cardiac enzymes, troponin
- Echocardiogram
- C R

Followup — Holter monitor

# Back Pain

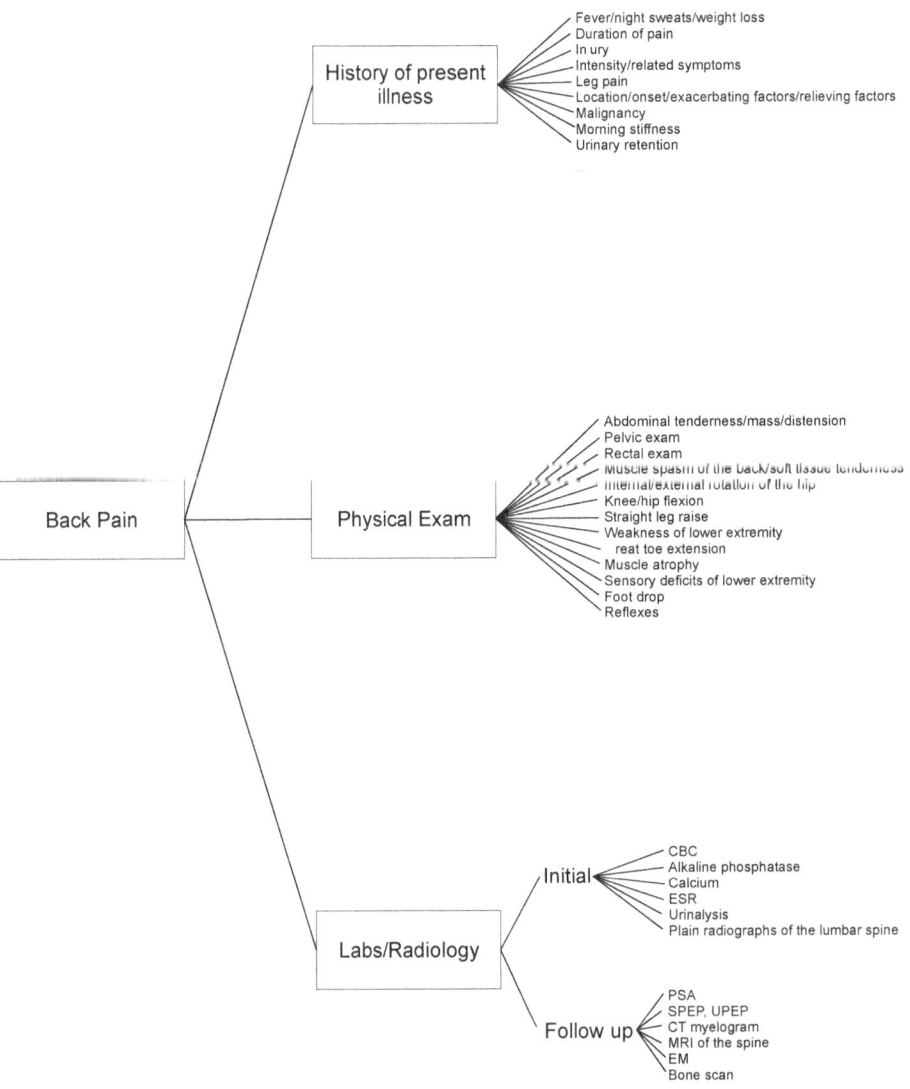

**History of present illness**
- Fever/night sweats/weight loss
- Duration of pain
- In ury
- Intensity/related symptoms
- Leg pain
- Location/onset/exacerbating factors/relieving factors
- Malignancy
- Morning stiffness
- Urinary retention

**Physical Exam**
- Abdominal tenderness/mass/distension
- Pelvic exam
- Rectal exam
- Muscle spasm of the back/soft tissue tenderness
- Internal/external rotation of the hip
- Knee/hip flexion
- Straight leg raise
- Weakness of lower extremity
- reat toe extension
- Muscle atrophy
- Sensory deficits of lower extremity
- Foot drop
- Reflexes

**Back Pain**

**Labs/Radiology**

Initial
- CBC
- Alkaline phosphatase
- Calcium
- ESR
- Urinalysis
- Plain radiographs of the lumbar spine

Follow up
- PSA
- SPEP, UPEP
- CT myelogram
- MRI of the spine
- EM
- Bone scan

# Back Pain

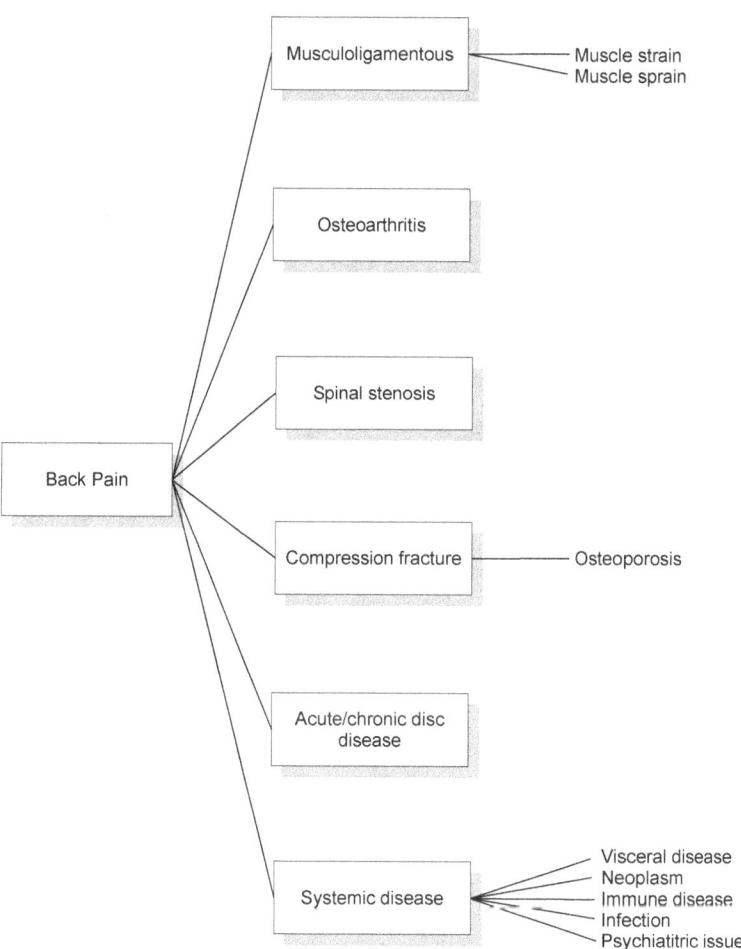

Reference: Deyo R Rainville J, Kent D. What can history and physical tell us about low back pain. JAMA.1992:268(6)760-5.

Andreili T, Bennett J, Carpenter C, Plum F, Smith L, Cecil Essentials of Medicine, ed 3, Philadelphia, 1993, W.B. Saunders Company. page 771

No Diagram for
this topic

# Congestive Heart Failure

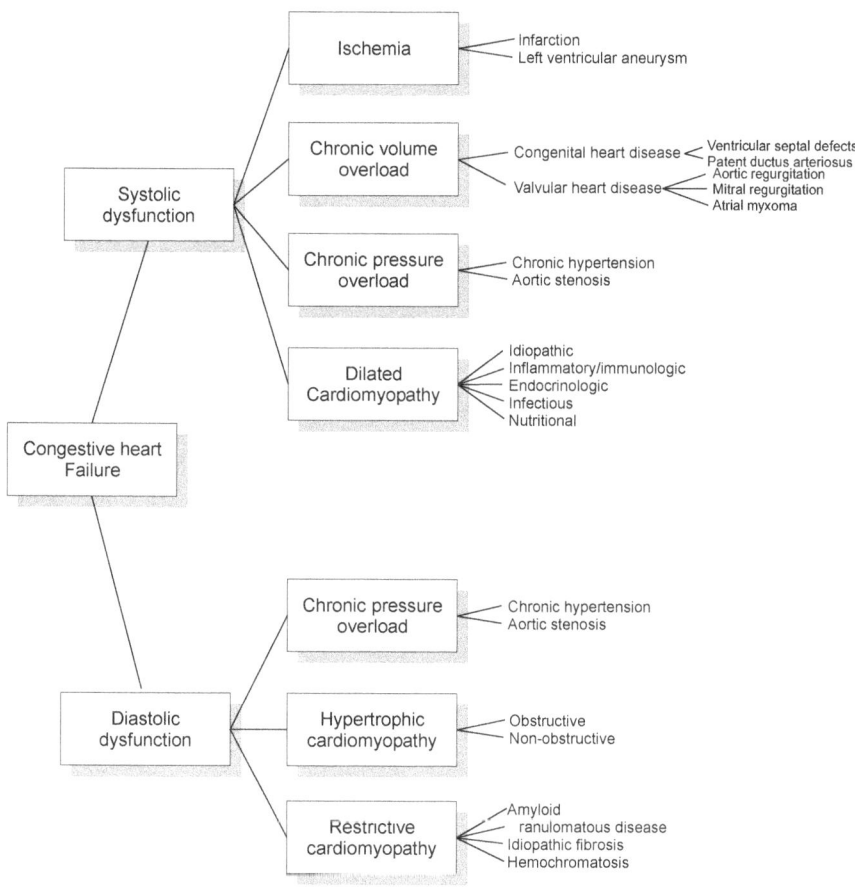

**Systolic dysfunction**
- Ischemia
  - Infarction
  - Left ventricular aneurysm
- Chronic volume overload
  - Congenital heart disease
    - Ventricular septal defects
    - Patent ductus arteriosus
  - Valvular heart disease
    - Aortic regurgitation
    - Mitral regurgitation
    - Atrial myxoma
- Chronic pressure overload
  - Chronic hypertension
  - Aortic stenosis
- Dilated Cardiomyopathy
  - Idiopathic
  - Inflammatory/immunologic
  - Endocrinologic
  - Infectious
  - Nutritional

**Congestive heart Failure**

**Diastolic dysfunction**
- Chronic pressure overload
  - Chronic hypertension
  - Aortic stenosis
- Hypertrophic cardiomyopathy
  - Obstructive
  - Non-obstructive
- Restrictive cardiomyopathy
  - Amyloid
  - ranulomatous disease
  - Idiopathic fibrosis
  - Hemochromatosis

Reference: Kelley, Essentials In Internal Medicine, ed 3. Philadelphia, 1994,J.B. Lippincott, page 78

Reference: Weinberger H. Diagnosis and treatment of diastolic heart failure. Hospital physician, March 15; 115-126,19998

# Congestive Heart Failure

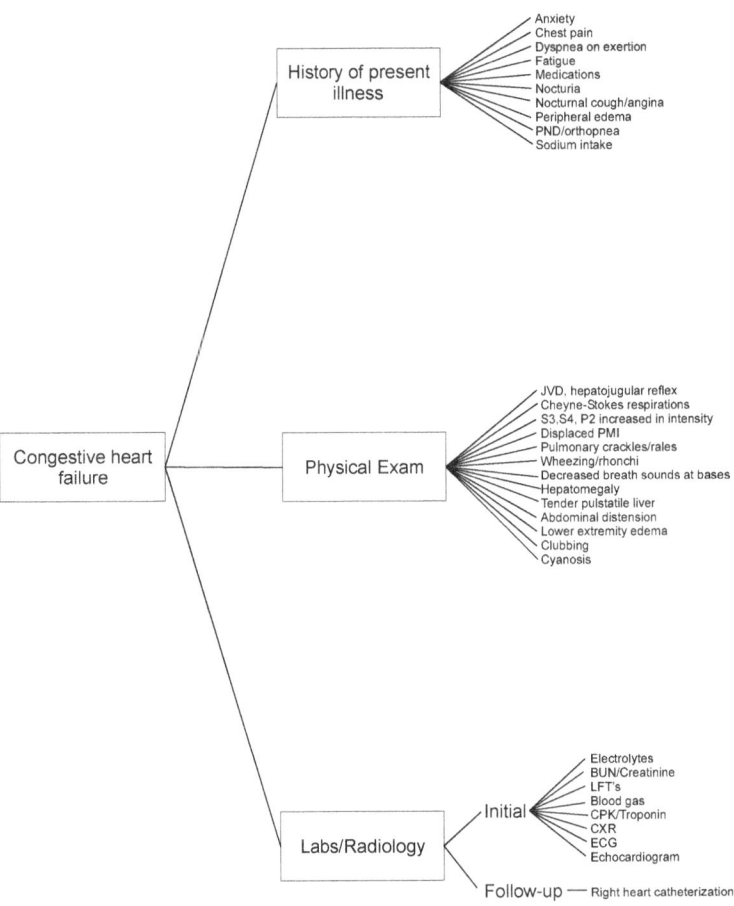

**History of present illness**
- Anxiety
- Chest pain
- Dyspnea on exertion
- Fatigue
- Medications
- Nocturia
- Nocturnal cough/angina
- Peripheral edema
- PND/orthopnea
- Sodium intake

**Congestive heart failure**

**Physical Exam**
- JVD, hepatojugular reflex
- Cheyne-Stokes respirations
- S3,S4, P2 increased in intensity
- Displaced PMI
- Pulmonary crackles/rales
- Wheezing/rhonchi
- Decreased breath sounds at bases
- Hepatomegaly
- Tender pulsatile liver
- Abdominal distension
- Lower extremity edema
- Clubbing
- Cyanosis

**Labs/Radiology**

Initial
- Electrolytes
- BUN/Creatinine
- LFT's
- Blood gas
- CPK/Troponin
- CXR
- ECG
- Echocardiogram

Follow-up — Right heart catheterization

# Chronic Cough

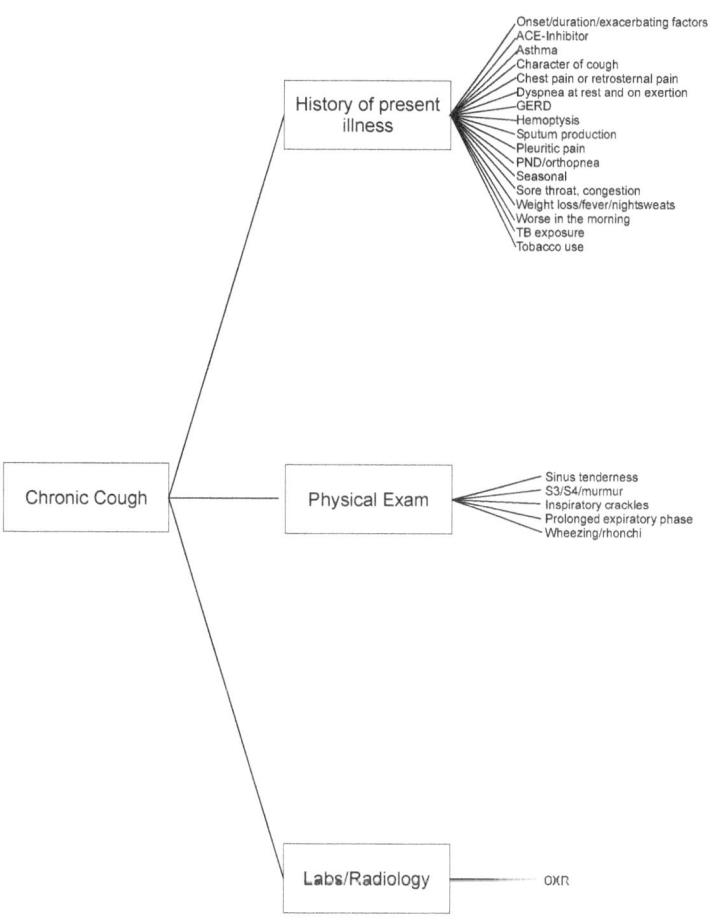

**Chronic Cough**

**History of present illness**
- Onset/duration/exacerbating factors
- ACE-Inhibitor
- Asthma
- Character of cough
- Chest pain or retrosternal pain
- Dyspnea at rest and on exertion
- GERD
- Hemoptysis
- Sputum production
- Pleuritic pain
- PND/orthopnea
- Seasonal
- Sore throat, congestion
- Weight loss/fever/nightsweats
- Worse in the morning
- TB exposure
- Tobacco use

**Physical Exam**
- Sinus tenderness
- S3/S4/murmur
- Inspiratory crackles
- Prolonged expiratory phase
- Wheezing/rhonchi

**Labs/Radiology**
- CXR

# Cirrhosis

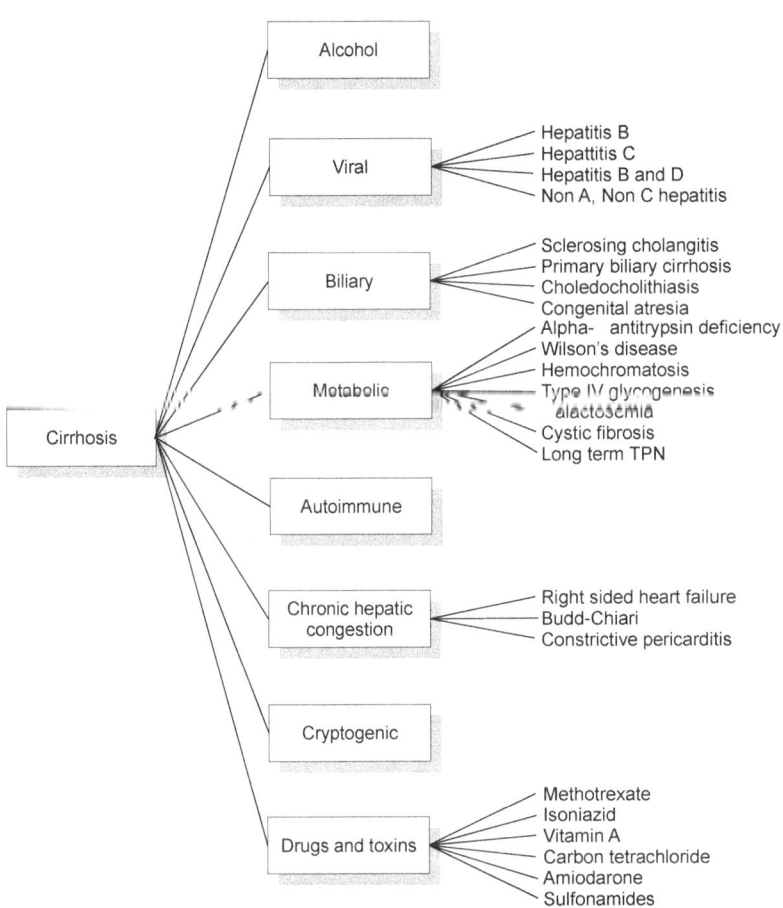

Alcohol

Viral
- Hepatitis B
- Hepattitis C
- Hepatitis B and D
- Non A, Non C hepatitis

Biliary
- Sclerosing cholangitis
- Primary biliary cirrhosis
- Choledocholithiasis
- Congenital atresia

Metabolic
- Alpha- antitrypsin deficiency
- Wilson's disease
- Hemochromatosis
- Type IV glycogenesis
- alactosemia
- Cystic fibrosis
- Long term TPN

Autoimmune

Chronic hepatic congestion
- Right sided heart failure
- Budd-Chiari
- Constrictive pericarditis

Cryptogenic

Drugs and toxins
- Methotrexate
- Isoniazid
- Vitamin A
- Carbon tetrachloride
- Amiodarone
- Sulfonamides

Cirrhosis

Mcguire B, Bloomer J. Complications of cirrhosis. Why they occur and what to do about them. Postgrad Med 1998;103(2):209-12, 217-8, 223-4.

# Cirrhosis

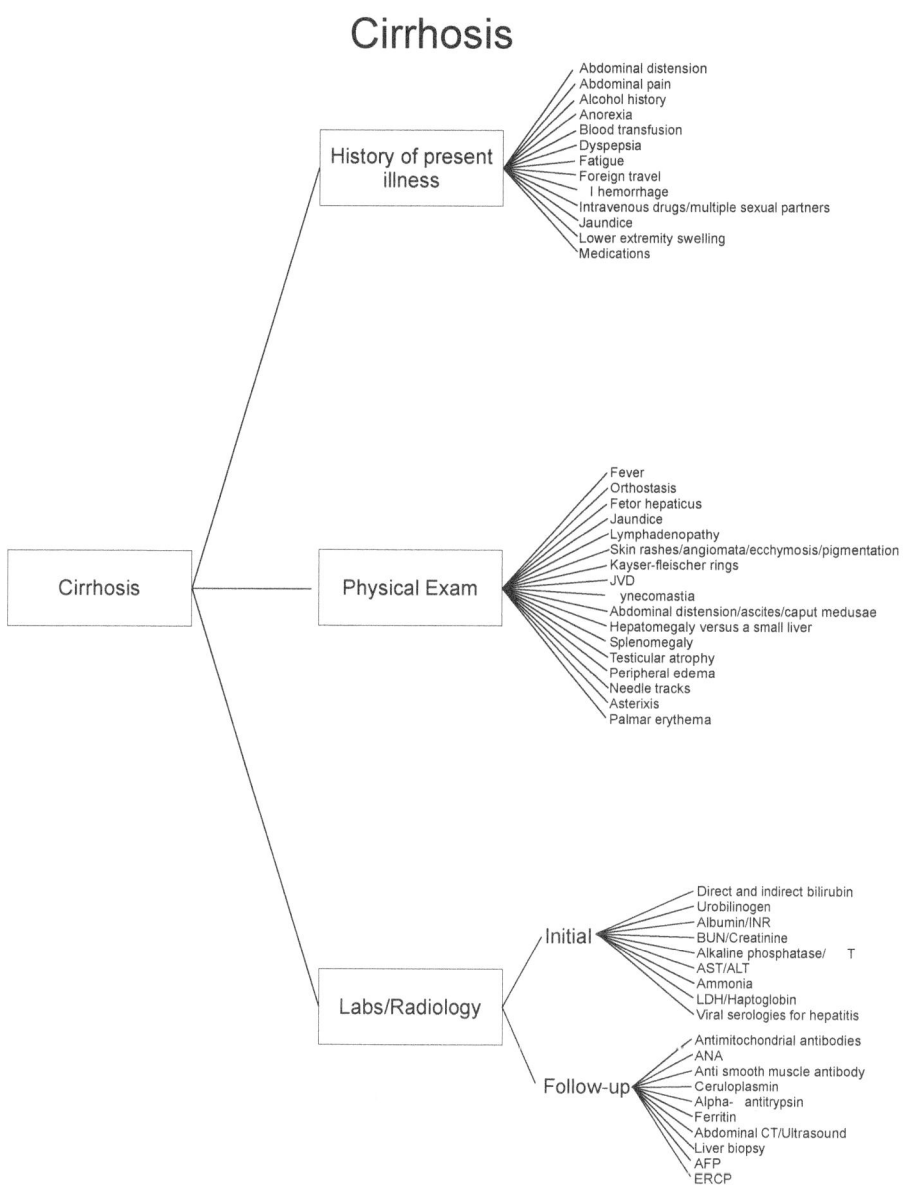

**Cirrhosis**

**History of present illness**
- Abdominal distension
- Abdominal pain
- Alcohol history
- Anorexia
- Blood transfusion
- Dyspepsia
- Fatigue
- Foreign travel
- I hemorrhage
- Intravenous drugs/multiple sexual partners
- Jaundice
- Lower extremity swelling
- Medications

**Physical Exam**
- Fever
- Orthostasis
- Fetor hepaticus
- Jaundice
- Lymphadenopathy
- Skin rashes/angiomata/ecchymosis/pigmentation
- Kayser-fleischer rings
- JVD
- ynecomastia
- Abdominal distension/ascites/caput medusae
- Hepatomegaly versus a small liver
- Splenomegaly
- Testicular atrophy
- Peripheral edema
- Needle tracks
- Asterixis
- Palmar erythema

**Labs/Radiology**

Initial
- Direct and indirect bilirubin
- Urobilinogen
- Albumin/INR
- BUN/Creatinine
- Alkaline phosphatase/    T
- AST/ALT
- Ammonia
- LDH/Haptoglobin
- Viral serologies for hepatitis

Follow-up
- Antimitochondrial antibodies
- ANA
- Anti smooth muscle antibody
- Ceruloplasmin
- Alpha- antitrypsin
- Ferritin
- Abdominal CT/Ultrasound
- Liver biopsy
- AFP
- ERCP

# Constipation

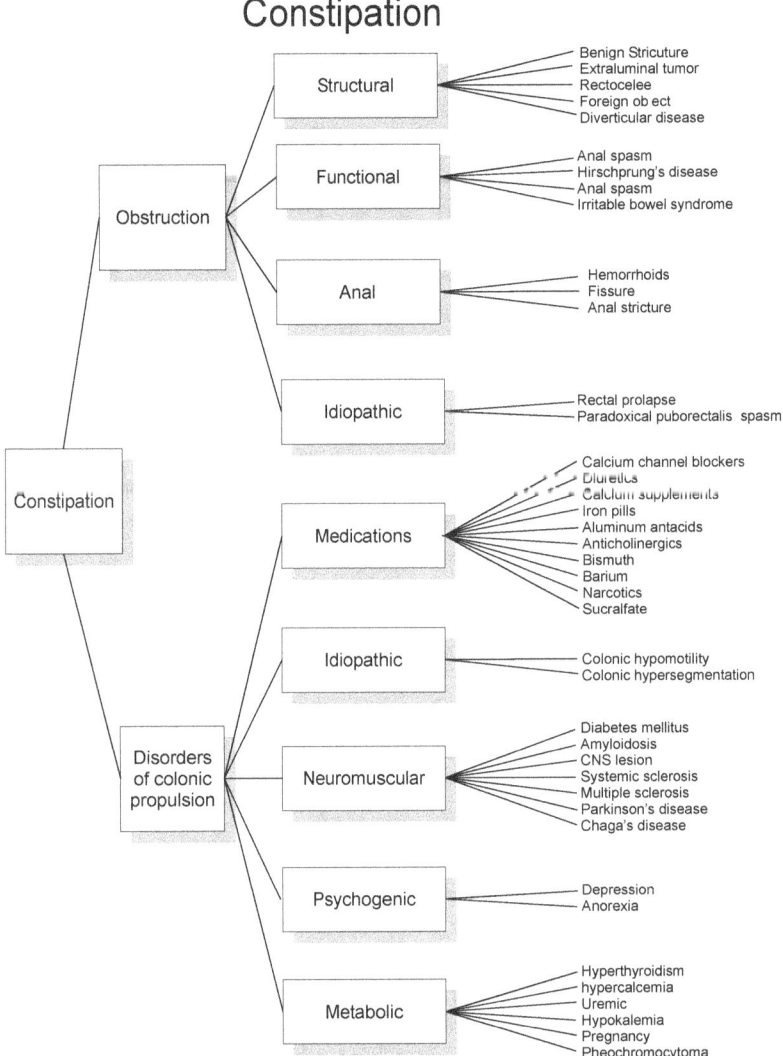

- Constipation
  - Obstruction
    - Structural
      - Benign Stricture
      - Extraluminal tumor
      - Rectocelee
      - Foreign ob ect
      - Diverticular disease
    - Functional
      - Anal spasm
      - Hirschprung's disease
      - Anal spasm
      - Irritable bowel syndrome
    - Anal
      - Hemorrhoids
      - Fissure
      - Anal stricture
    - Idiopathic
      - Rectal prolapse
      - Paradoxical puborectalis  spasm
  - Disorders of colonic propulsion
    - Medications
      - Calcium channel blockers
      - Diuretics
      - Calcium supplements
      - Iron pills
      - Aluminum antacids
      - Anticholinergics
      - Bismuth
      - Barium
      - Narcotics
      - Sucralfate
    - Idiopathic
      - Colonic hypomotility
      - Colonic hypersegmentation
    - Neuromuscular
      - Diabetes mellitus
      - Amyloidosis
      - CNS lesion
      - Systemic sclerosis
      - Multiple sclerosis
      - Parkinson's disease
      - Chaga's disease
    - Psychogenic
      - Depression
      - Anorexia
    - Metabolic
      - Hyperthyroidism
      - hypercalcemia
      - Uremic
      - Hypokalemia
      - Pregnancy
      - Pheochromocytoma

Reference  Thompson W, Longstreth  , Drossman D  Functional bowel disorders and functional abdominal pain    ut    4  Suppl 2 Il43-

# Constipation

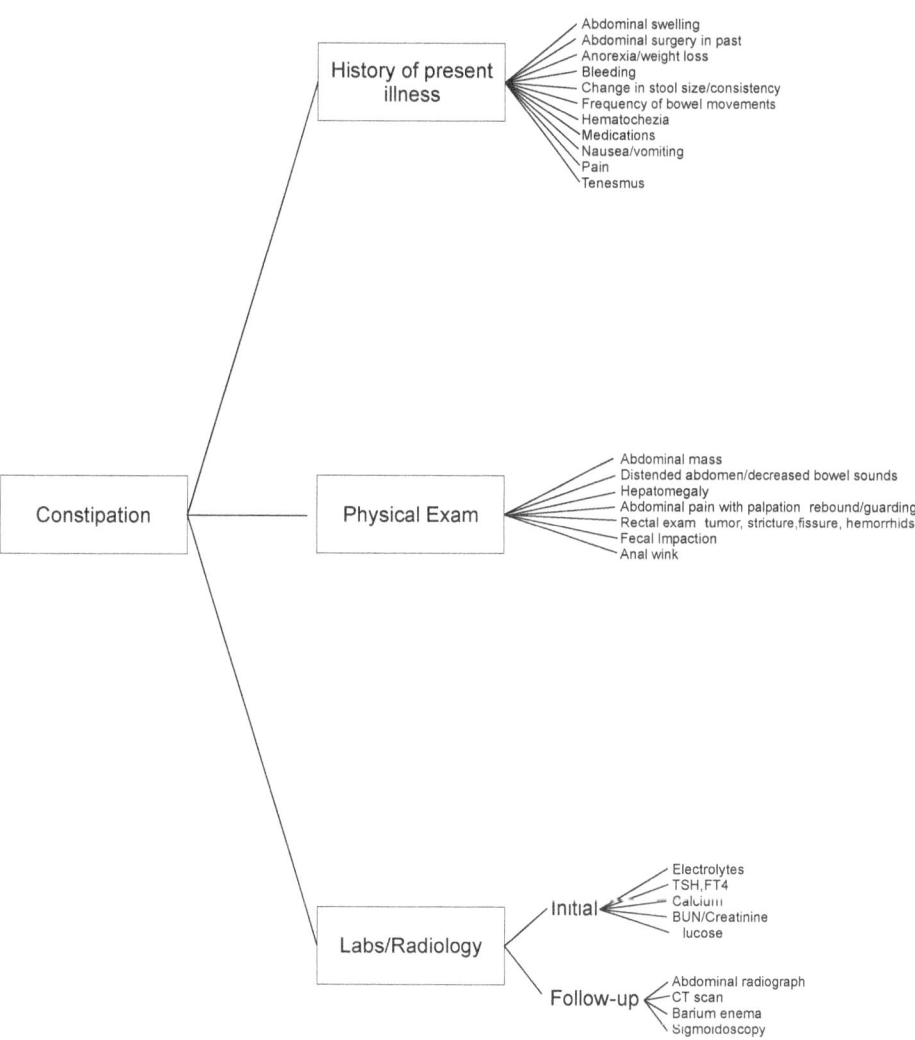

**History of present illness**
- Abdominal swelling
- Abdominal surgery in past
- Anorexia/weight loss
- Bleeding
- Change in stool size/consistency
- Frequency of bowel movements
- Hematochezia
- Medications
- Nausea/vomiting
- Pain
- Tenesmus

**Physical Exam**
- Abdominal mass
- Distended abdomen/decreased bowel sounds
- Hepatomegaly
- Abdominal pain with palpation  rebound/guarding
- Rectal exam  tumor, stricture,fissure, hemorrhids
- Fecal Impaction
- Anal wink

**Labs/Radiology**

Initial
- Electrolytes
- TSH,FT4
- Calcium
- BUN/Creatinine
- lucose

Follow-up
- Abdominal radiograph
- CT scan
- Barium enema
- Sigmoidoscopy

# Chronic Cough

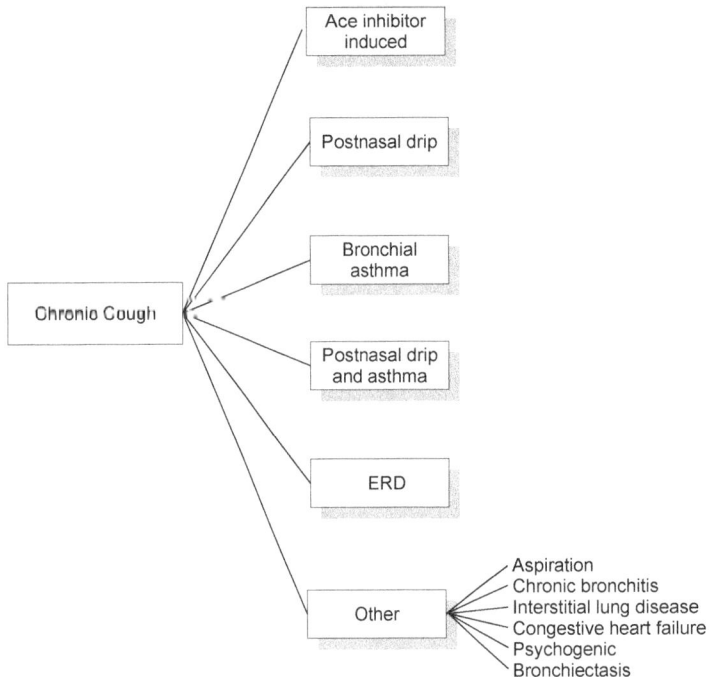

Reference  Tan R, Spector S  Chronic cough  Comprehensive therapy    23    4    -

# Diabetes Insipidus

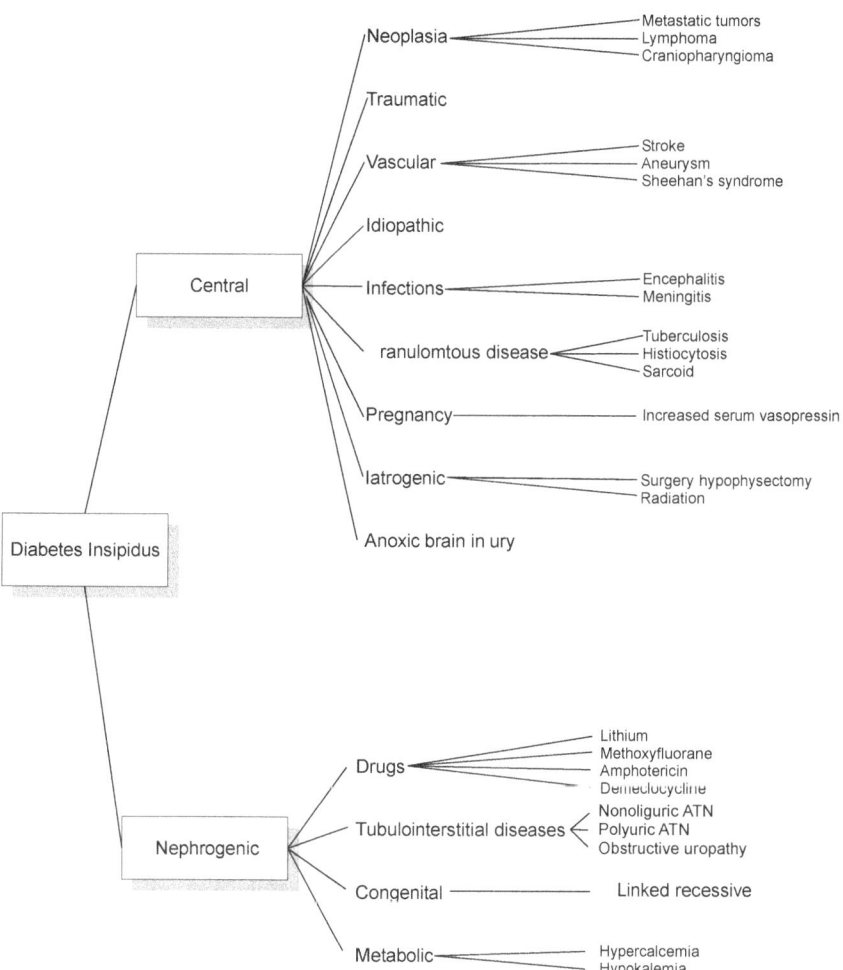

Reference: Singer I, Oster J, Fishman L. The management of diabetes insipidus in adults. Arch Intern Med 1997;157(12):1293-301.

# Diabetes Insipidus

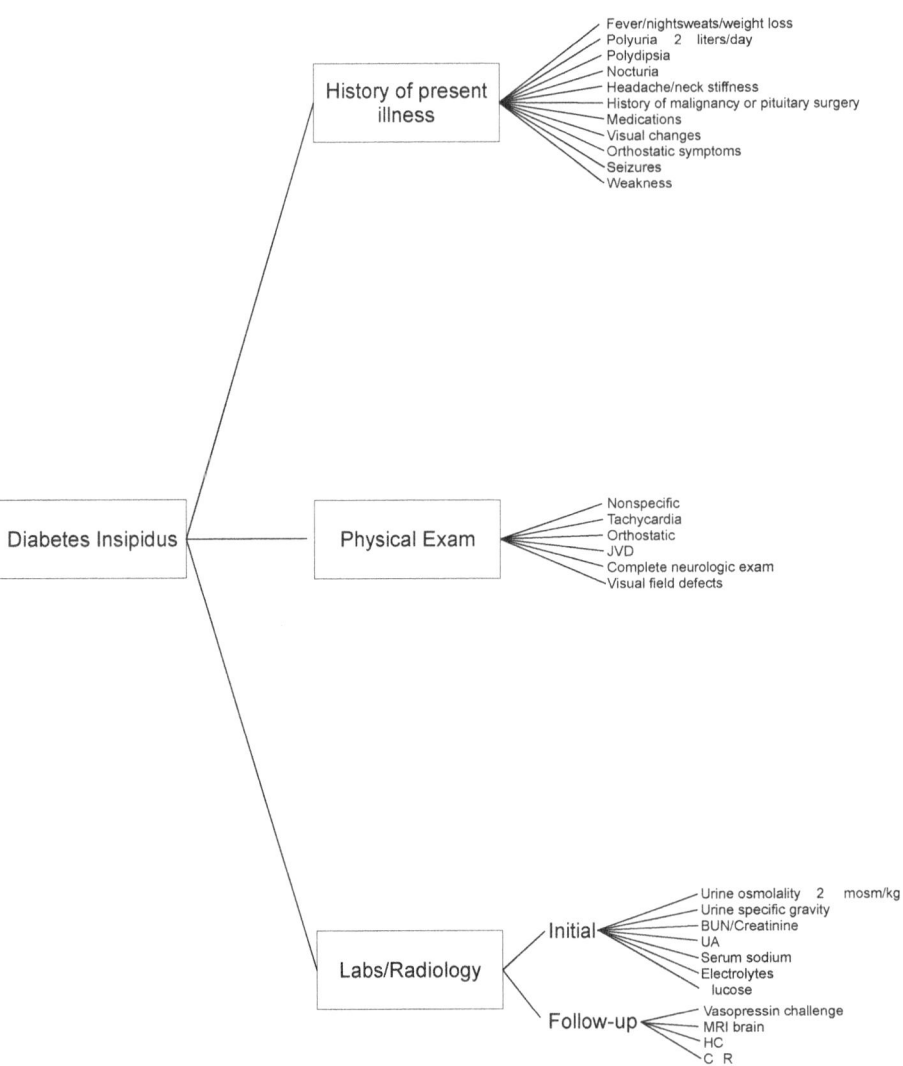

**History of present illness**
- Fever/nightsweats/weight loss
- Polyuria 2 liters/day
- Polydipsia
- Nocturia
- Headache/neck stiffness
- History of malignancy or pituitary surgery
- Medications
- Visual changes
- Orthostatic symptoms
- Seizures
- Weakness

**Physical Exam**
- Nonspecific
- Tachycardia
- Orthostatic
- JVD
- Complete neurologic exam
- Visual field defects

**Labs/Radiology**

Initial
- Urine osmolality 2 mosm/kg
- Urine specific gravity
- BUN/Creatinine
- UA
- Serum sodium
- Electrolytes
- lucose

Follow-up
- Vasopressin challenge
- MRI brain
- HC
- C R

# Diarrhea (Chronic)

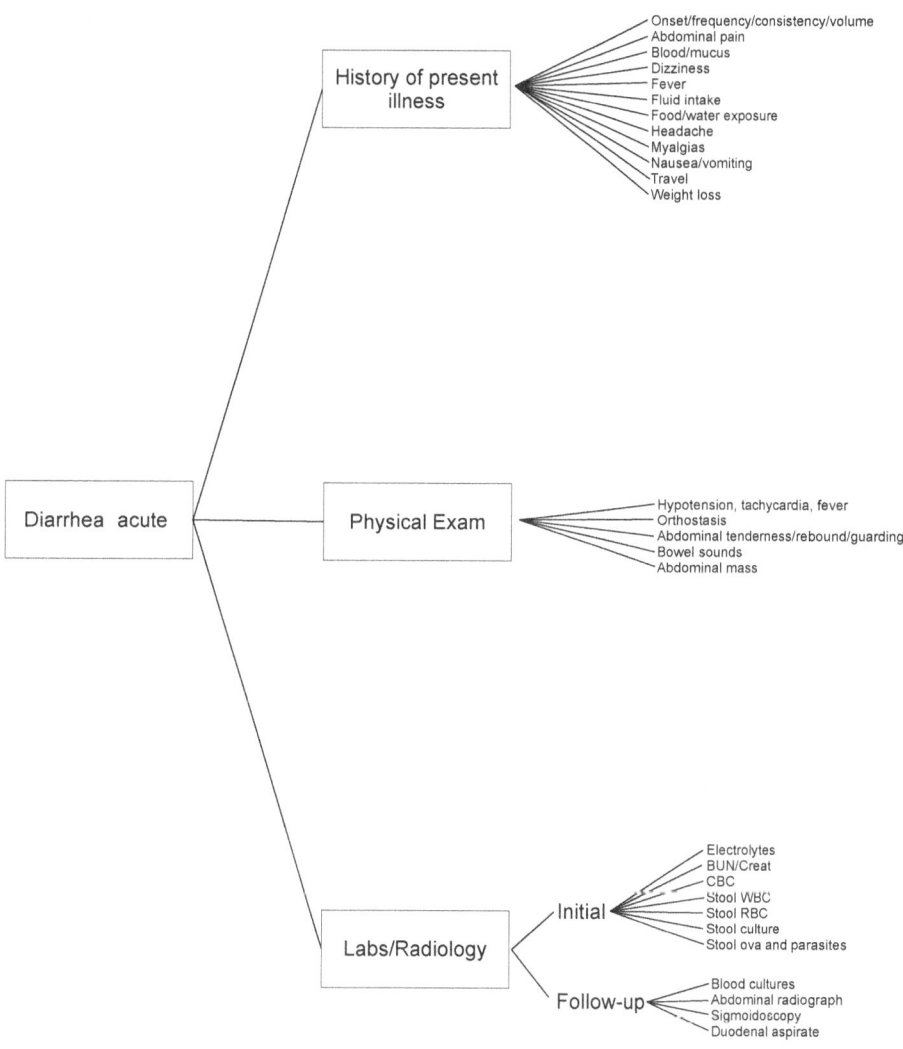

**History of present illness**
- Onset/frequency/consistency/volume
- Abdominal pain
- Blood/mucus
- Dizziness
- Fever
- Fluid intake
- Food/water exposure
- Headache
- Myalgias
- Nausea/vomiting
- Travel
- Weight loss

**Diarrhea acute**

**Physical Exam**
- Hypotension, tachycardia, fever
- Orthostasis
- Abdominal tenderness/rebound/guarding
- Bowel sounds
- Abdominal mass

**Labs/Radiology**

Initial
- Electrolytes
- BUN/Creat
- CBC
- Stool WBC
- Stool RBC
- Stool culture
- Stool ova and parasites

Follow-up
- Blood cultures
- Abdominal radiograph
- Sigmoidoscopy
- Duodenal aspirate

# Infectious Diarrhea

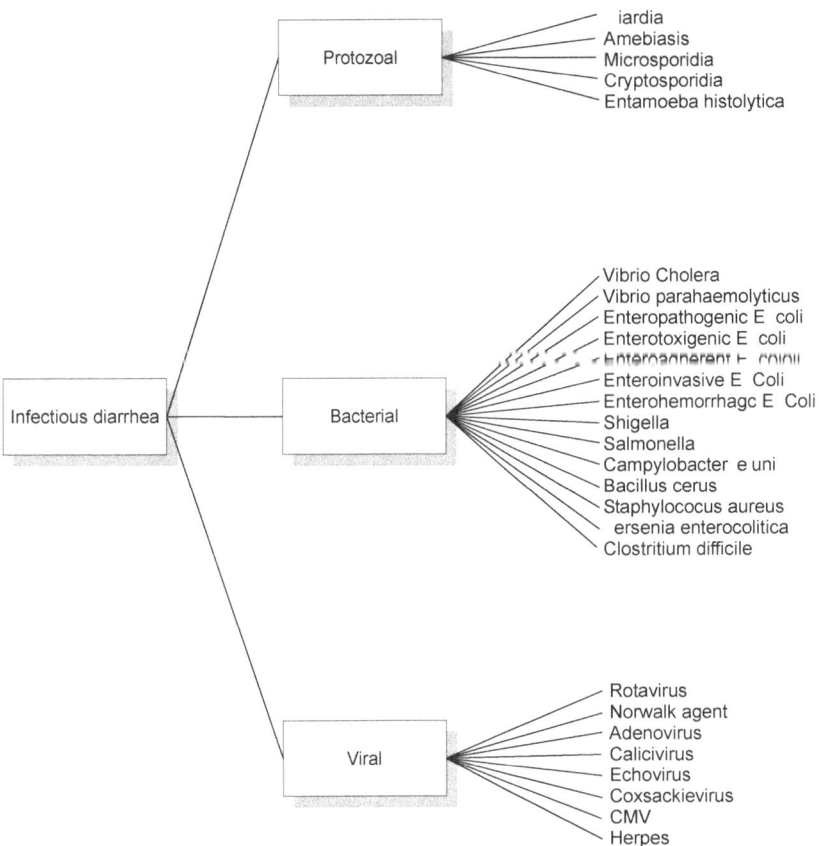

Protozoal
- iardia
- Amebiasis
- Microsporidia
- Cryptosporidia
- Entamoeba histolytica

Bacterial
- Vibrio Cholera
- Vibrio parahaemolyticus
- Enteropathogenic E coli
- Enterotoxigenic E coli
- Enteroadherent E coini
- Enteroinvasive E Coli
- Enterohemorrhagc E Coli
- Shigella
- Salmonella
- Campylobacter e uni
- Bacillus cerus
- Staphylococus aureus
- ersenia enterocolitica
- Clostritium difficile

Viral
- Rotavirus
- Norwalk agent
- Adenovirus
- Calicivirus
- Echovirus
- Coxsackievirus
- CMV
- Herpes

Infectious diarrhea

Reference:Sutjita M, Dupont H, Guidelines on acute infectious diarrhea in adults: the practice parameters committee of the american college of gastroenterology.1997;92:1962-1975
Andreili T, Bennett J, Carpenter C, Plum F, Smith L, Cecil Essentials of Medicine, ed 3, Philadelphia, 1993, W.B. Saunders Company. page 6

# Dizziness

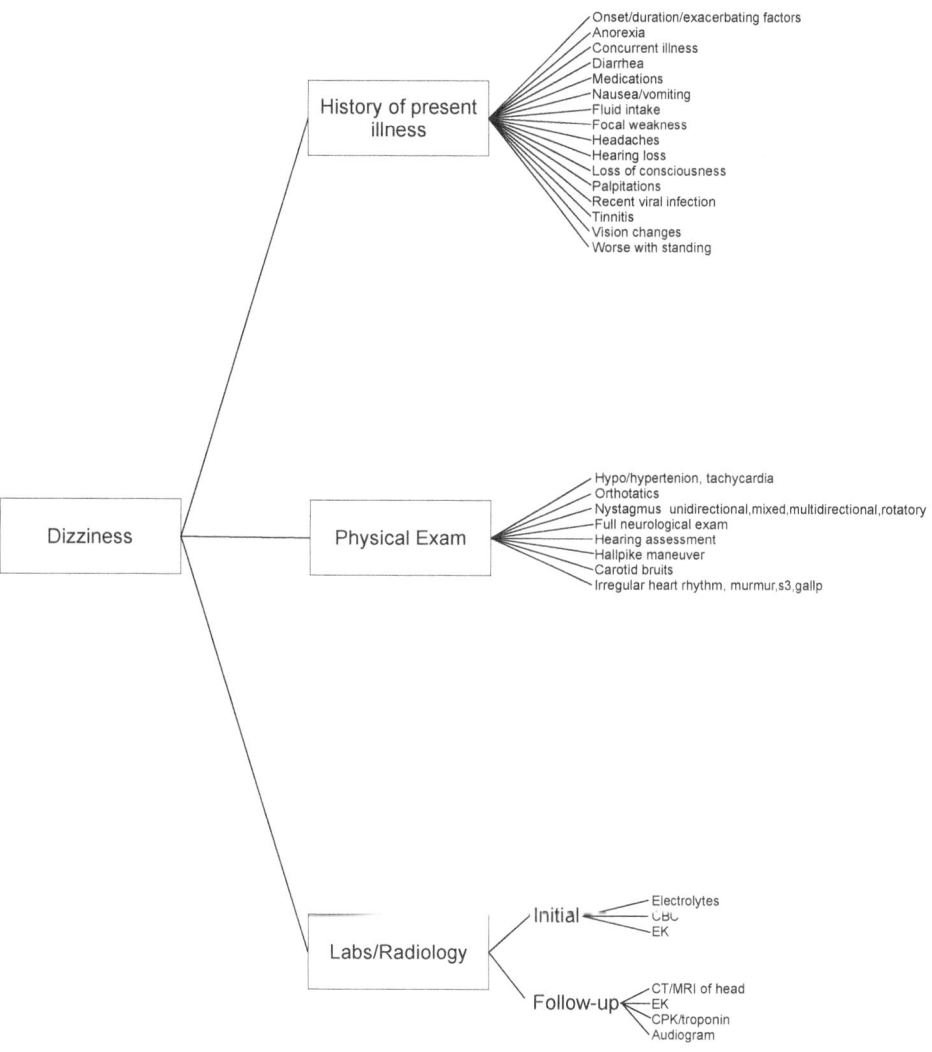

**History of present illness**
- Onset/duration/exacerbating factors
- Anorexia
- Concurrent illness
- Diarrhea
- Medications
- Nausea/vomiting
- Fluid intake
- Focal weakness
- Headaches
- Hearing loss
- Loss of consciousness
- Palpitations
- Recent viral infection
- Tinnitis
- Vision changes
- Worse with standing

**Physical Exam**
- Hypo/hypertenion, tachycardia
- Orthotatics
- Nystagmus  unidirectional,mixed,multidirectional,rotatory
- Full neurological exam
- Hearing assessment
- Hallpike maneuver
- Carotid bruits
- Irregular heart rhythm, murmur,s3,gallp

**Labs/Radiology**
- Initial
  - Electrolytes
  - CBC
  - EK
- Follow-up
  - CT/MRI of head
  - EK
  - CPK/troponin
  - Audiogram

# Dizziness

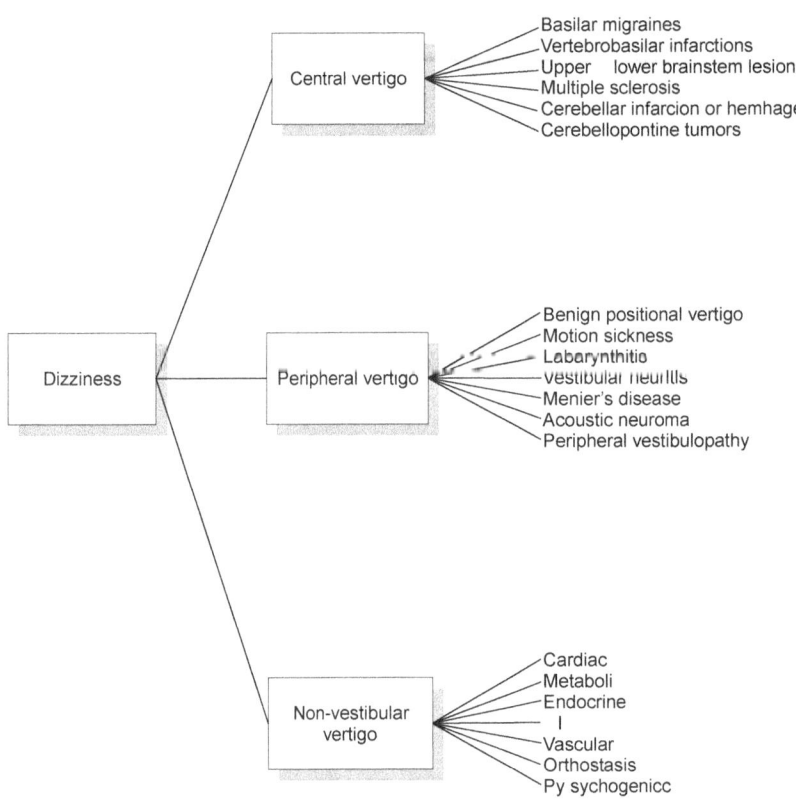

**Central vertigo**
- Basilar migraines
- Vertebrobasilar infarctions
- Upper   lower brainstem lesions
- Multiple sclerosis
- Cerebellar infarcion or hemhage
- Cerebellopontine tumors

**Dizziness**

**Peripheral vertigo**
- Benign positional vertigo
- Motion sickness
- Labarynthitia
- vestibular neuritis
- Menier's disease
- Acoustic neuroma
- Peripheral vestibulopathy

**Non-vestibular vertigo**
- Cardiac
- Metaboli
- Endocrine
- I
- Vascular
- Orthostasis
- Py sychogenicc

Baloh R. The dizzy patient. Postgraduate Medicine;1999;105(2);161-172.
Reference: Walker J, Barnes B. Dizzyness, Emergency medicine clinics of North America, 1998;16(4);845-875

# Dysphagia

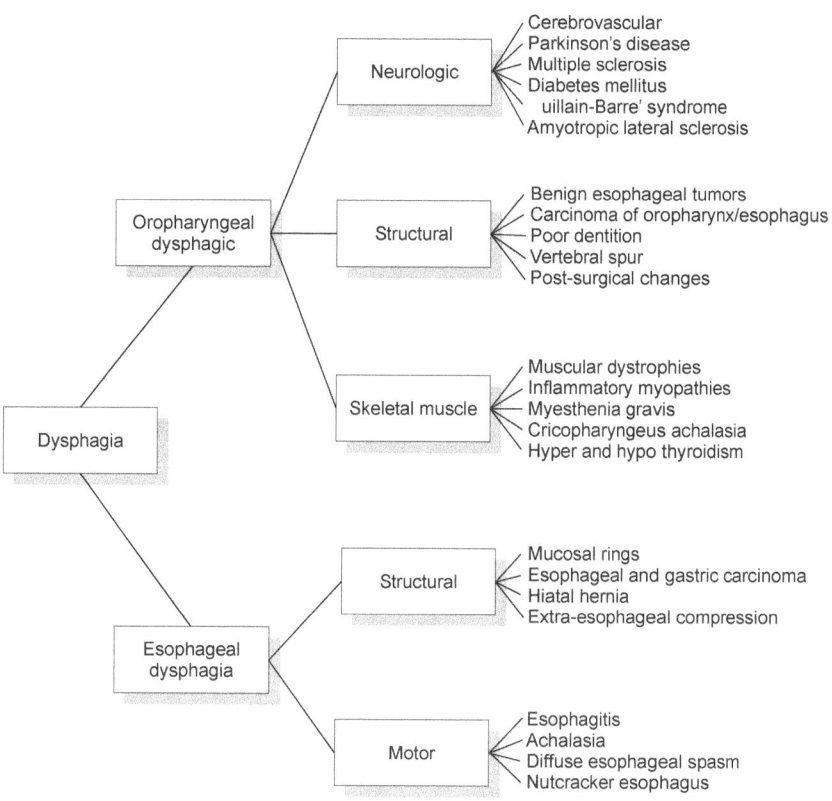

Neurologic
- Cerebrovascular
- Parkinson's disease
- Multiple sclerosis
- Diabetes mellitus
- uillain-Barre' syndrome
- Amyotropic lateral sclerosis

Structural
- Benign esophageal tumors
- Carcinoma of oropharynx/esophagus
- Poor dentition
- Vertebral spur
- Post-surgical changes

Skeletal muscle
- Muscular dystrophies
- Inflammatory myopathies
- Myesthenia gravis
- Cricopharyngeus achalasia
- Hyper and hypo thyroidism

Structural
- Mucosal rings
- Esophageal and gastric carcinoma
- Hiatal hernia
- Extra-esophageal compression

Motor
- Esophagitis
- Achalasia
- Diffuse esophageal spasm
- Nutcracker esophagus

Oropharyngeal dysphagic

Dysphagia

Esophageal dysphagia

Reference: Barloon J, Bergus G, Lu C. Diagnostic imaging in the evaluation of dysphagia. American family physician 1996;53:535-546.

Andreili T, Bennett J, Carpenter C, Plum F, Smith L, Cecil Essentials of Medicine, ed 3, Philadelphia, 1993, W.B. Saunders Company. page 28

# Dysphagia

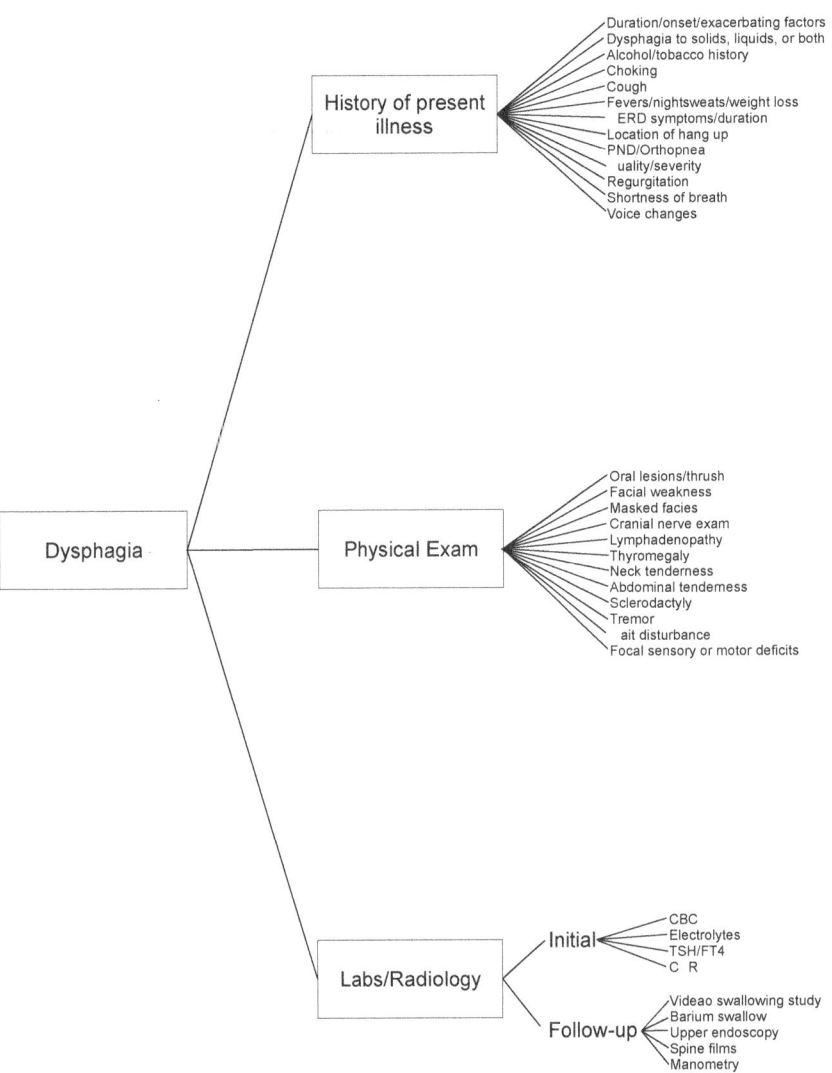

**Dysphagia**

**History of present illness**
- Duration/onset/exacerbating factors
- Dysphagia to solids, liquids, or both
- Alcohol/tobacco history
- Choking
- Cough
- Fevers/nightsweats/weight loss
- ERD symptoms/duration
- Location of hang up
- PND/Orthopnea
- uality/severity
- Regurgitation
- Shortness of breath
- Voice changes

**Physical Exam**
- Oral lesions/thrush
- Facial weakness
- Masked facies
- Cranial nerve exam
- Lymphadenopathy
- Thyromegaly
- Neck tenderness
- Abdominal tenderness
- Sclerodactyly
- Tremor
- ait disturbance
- Focal sensory or motor deficits

**Labs/Radiology**

Initial
- CBC
- Electrolytes
- TSH/FT4
- C R

Follow-up
- Videao swallowing study
- Barium swallow
- Upper endoscopy
- Spine films
- Manometry

# Dyspnea  Acute

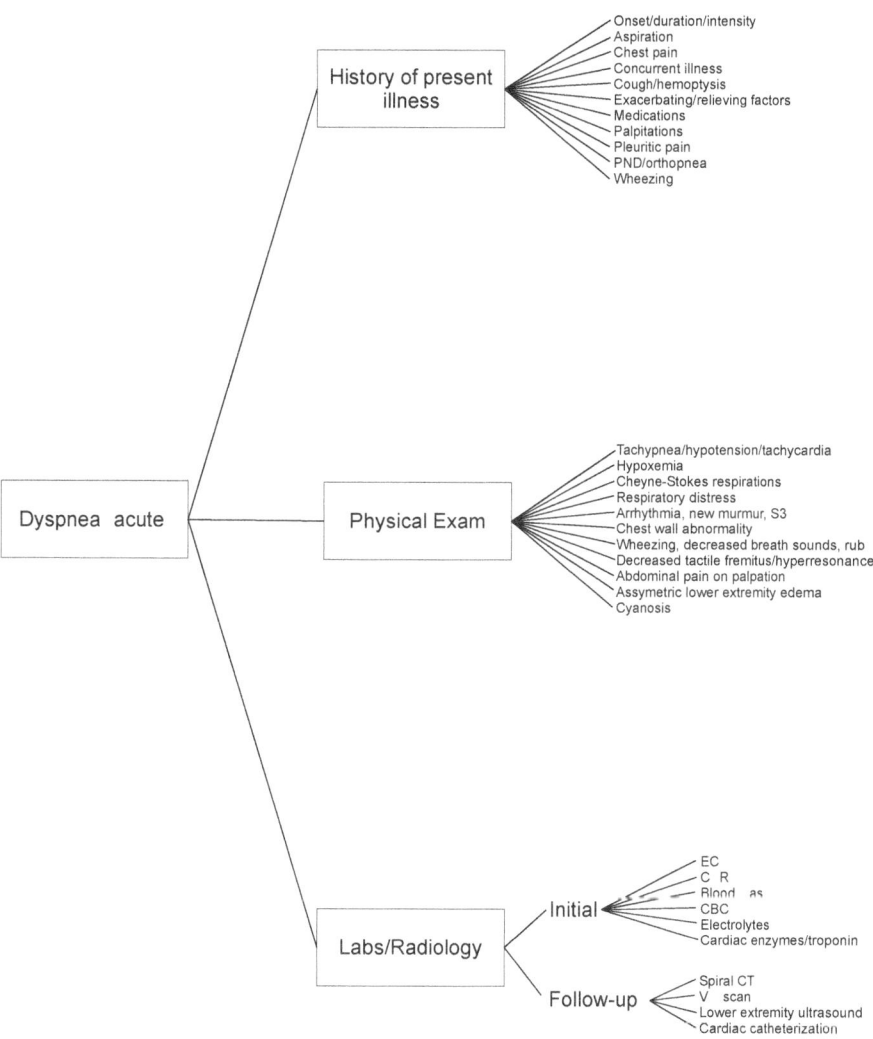

History of present illness
- Onset/duration/intensity
- Aspiration
- Chest pain
- Concurrent illness
- Cough/hemoptysis
- Exacerbating/relieving factors
- Medications
- Palpitations
- Pleuritic pain
- PND/orthopnea
- Wheezing

Dyspnea  acute

Physical Exam
- Tachypnea/hypotension/tachycardia
- Hypoxemia
- Cheyne-Stokes respirations
- Respiratory distress
- Arrhythmia, new murmur, S3
- Chest wall abnormality
- Wheezing, decreased breath sounds, rub
- Decreased tactile fremitus/hyperresonance
- Abdominal pain on palpation
- Assymetric lower extremity edema
- Cyanosis

Labs/Radiology

Initial
- EC
- C R
- Blood  as
- CBC
- Electrolytes
- Cardiac enzymes/troponin

Follow-up
- Spiral CT
- V  scan
- Lower extremity ultrasound
- Cardiac catheterization

# Acute Dyspnea

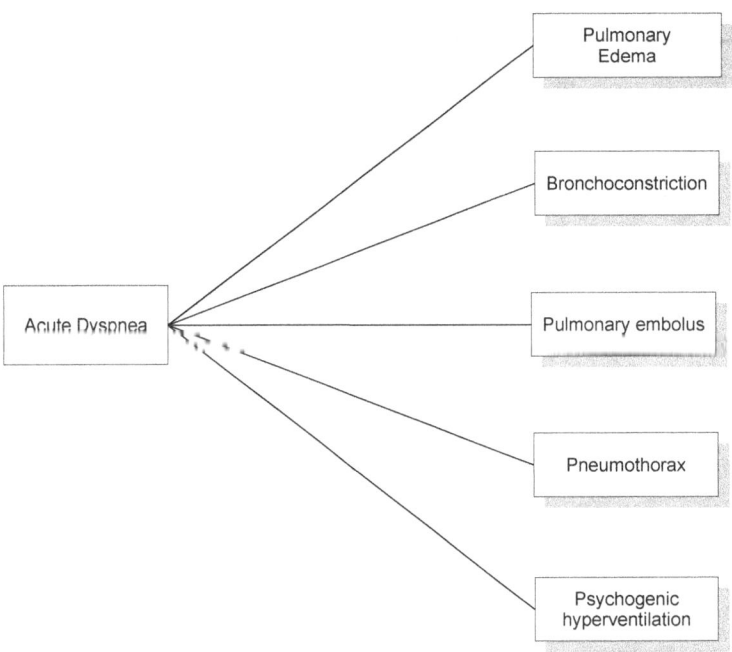

Weisman I, Zeballos R. Clinical evaluation of unexplained dyspnea. Cardiologia 1996;41(7):621-34.

# Eosinophilia

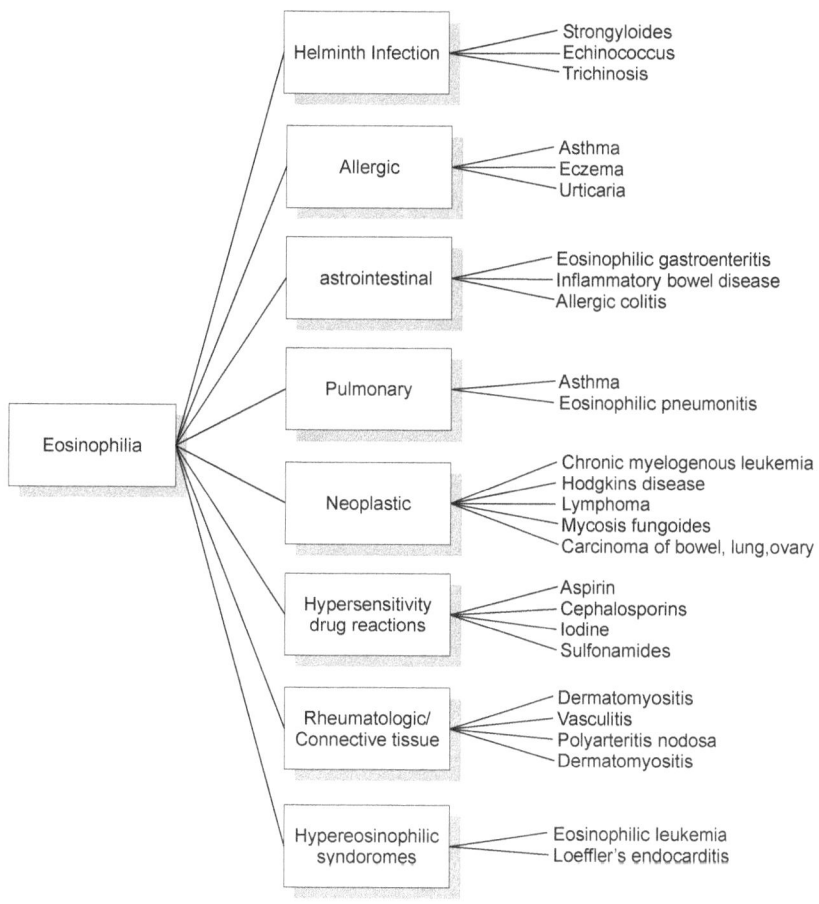

**Eosinophilia**

- **Helminth Infection**
  - Strongyloides
  - Echinococcus
  - Trichinosis

- **Allergic**
  - Asthma
  - Eczema
  - Urticaria

- **astrointestinal**
  - Eosinophilic gastroenteritis
  - Inflammatory bowel disease
  - Allergic colitis

- **Pulmonary**
  - Asthma
  - Eosinophilic pneumonitis

- **Neoplastic**
  - Chronic myelogenous leukemia
  - Hodgkins disease
  - Lymphoma
  - Mycosis fungoides
  - Carcinoma of bowel, lung, ovary

- **Hypersensitivity drug reactions**
  - Aspirin
  - Cephalosporins
  - Iodine
  - Sulfonamides

- **Rheumatologic/ Connective tissue**
  - Dermatomyositis
  - Vasculitis
  - Polyarteritis nodosa
  - Dermatomyositis

- **Hypereosinophilic syndoromes**
  - Eosinophilic leukemia
  - Loeffler's endocarditis

Reference: Bain B, Hypereosinophilia. Curr Opin Hematol 2000;7(1):21-5.

# Eosinophilia

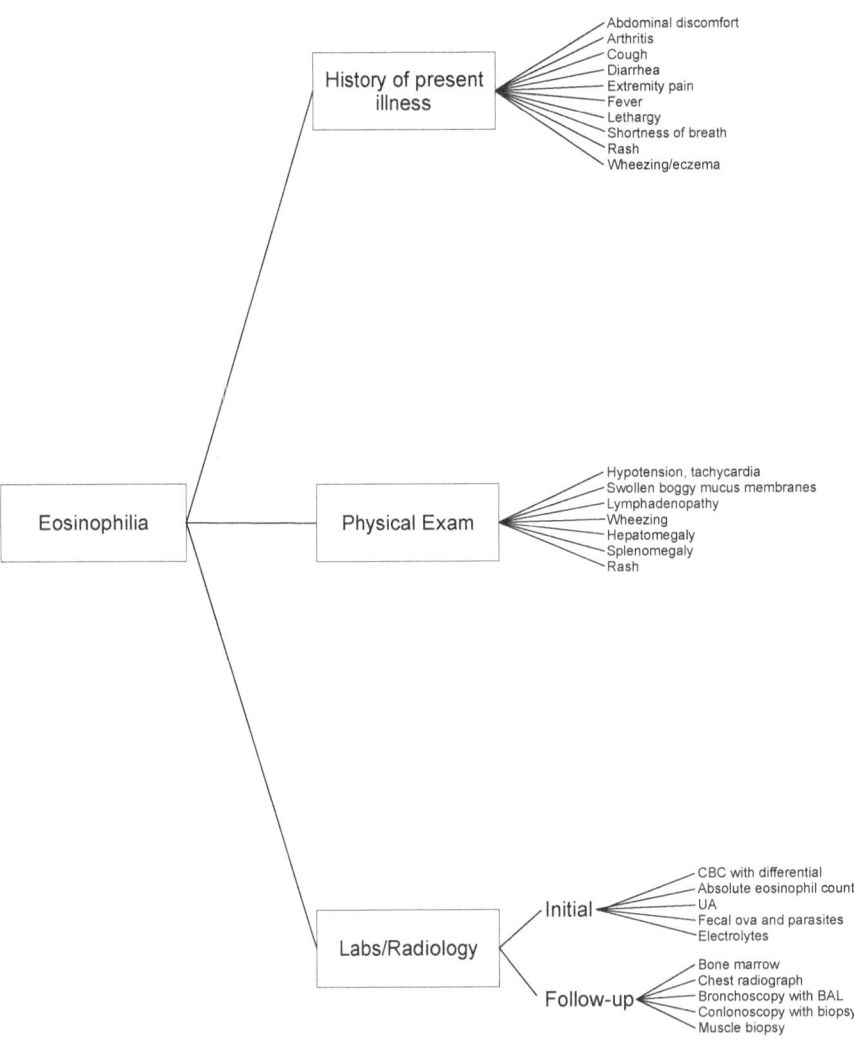

**History of present illness**
- Abdominal discomfort
- Arthritis
- Cough
- Diarrhea
- Extremity pain
- Fever
- Lethargy
- Shortness of breath
- Rash
- Wheezing/eczema

**Eosinophilia**

**Physical Exam**
- Hypotension, tachycardia
- Swollen boggy mucus membranes
- Lymphadenopathy
- Wheezing
- Hepatomegaly
- Splenomegaly
- Rash

**Labs/Radiology**

Initial
- CBC with differential
- Absolute eosinophil count
- UA
- Fecal ova and parasites
- Electrolytes

Follow-up
- Bone marrow
- Chest radiograph
- Bronchoscopy with BAL
- Conlonoscopy with biopsy
- Muscle biopsy

# alactorrhea

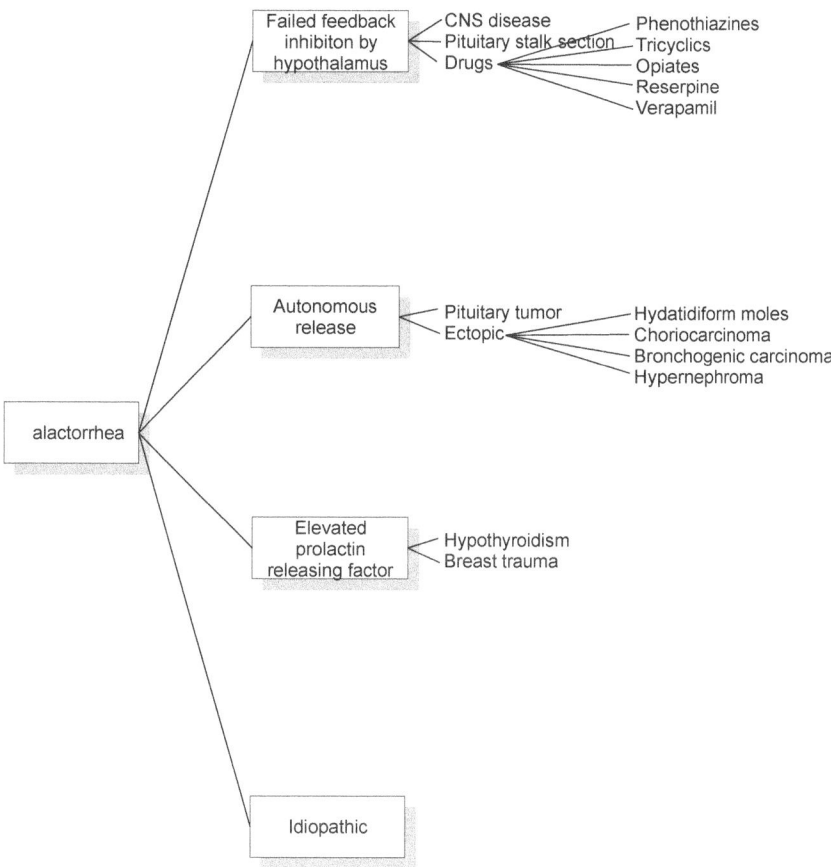

Reference: Haney A. Galactorrhea. Curr Ther Endocrinol Metab 1997;6:393-6.

# ynecomastia

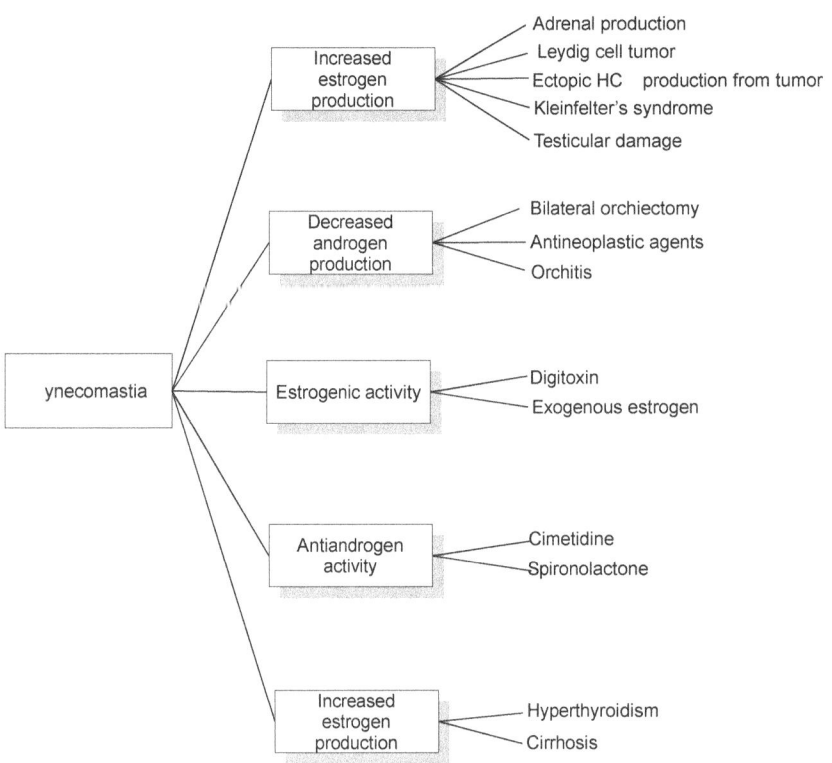

Neuman J. Evaluation and treatement of gynecomastia. Am Fam Physician 1997;55(5):1835-44,1849-50.

# Gynecomastia

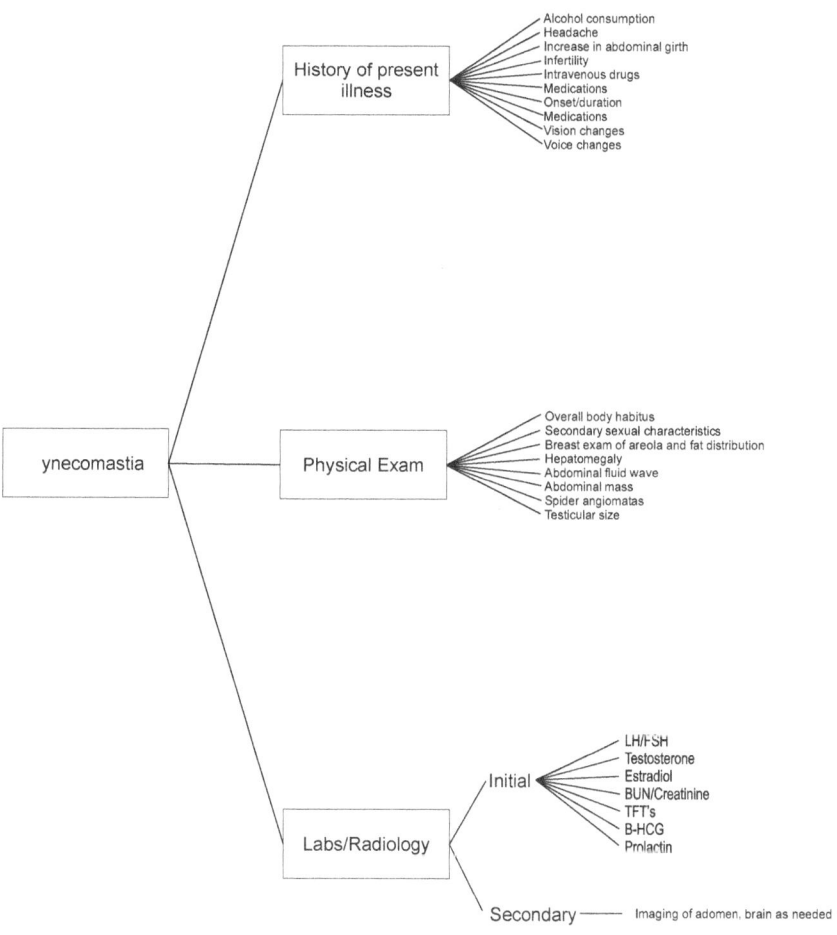

# Headache

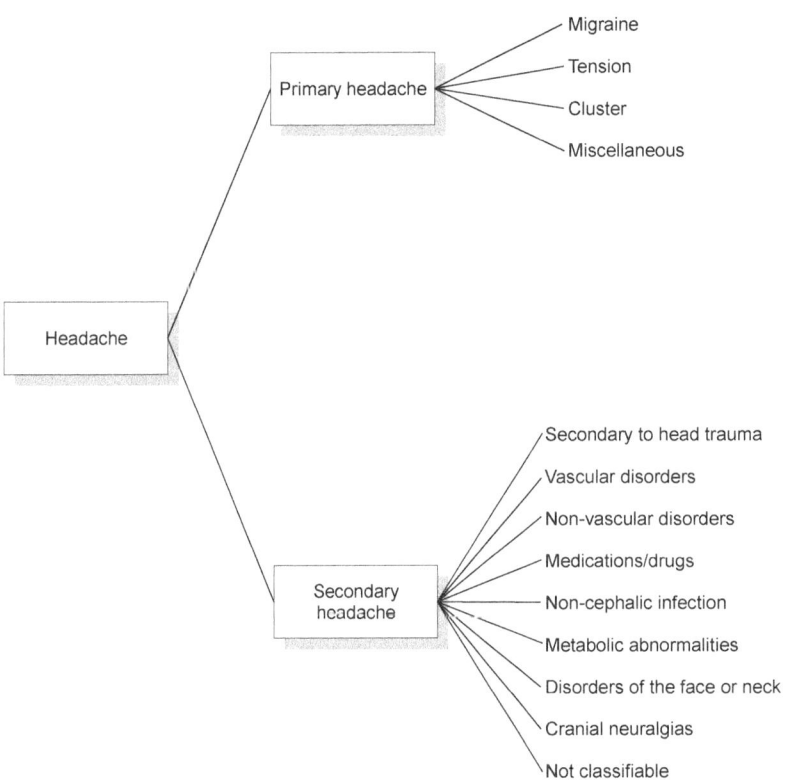

Primary headache
- Migraine
- Tension
- Cluster
- Miscellaneous

Secondary headache
- Secondary to head trauma
- Vascular disorders
- Non-vascular disorders
- Medications/drugs
- Non-cephalic infection
- Metabolic abnormalities
- Disorders of the face or neck
- Cranial neuralgias
- Not classifiable

Lipton RB Classification and epidemiology of headache - Clin Cornerstone -          -

# Headache

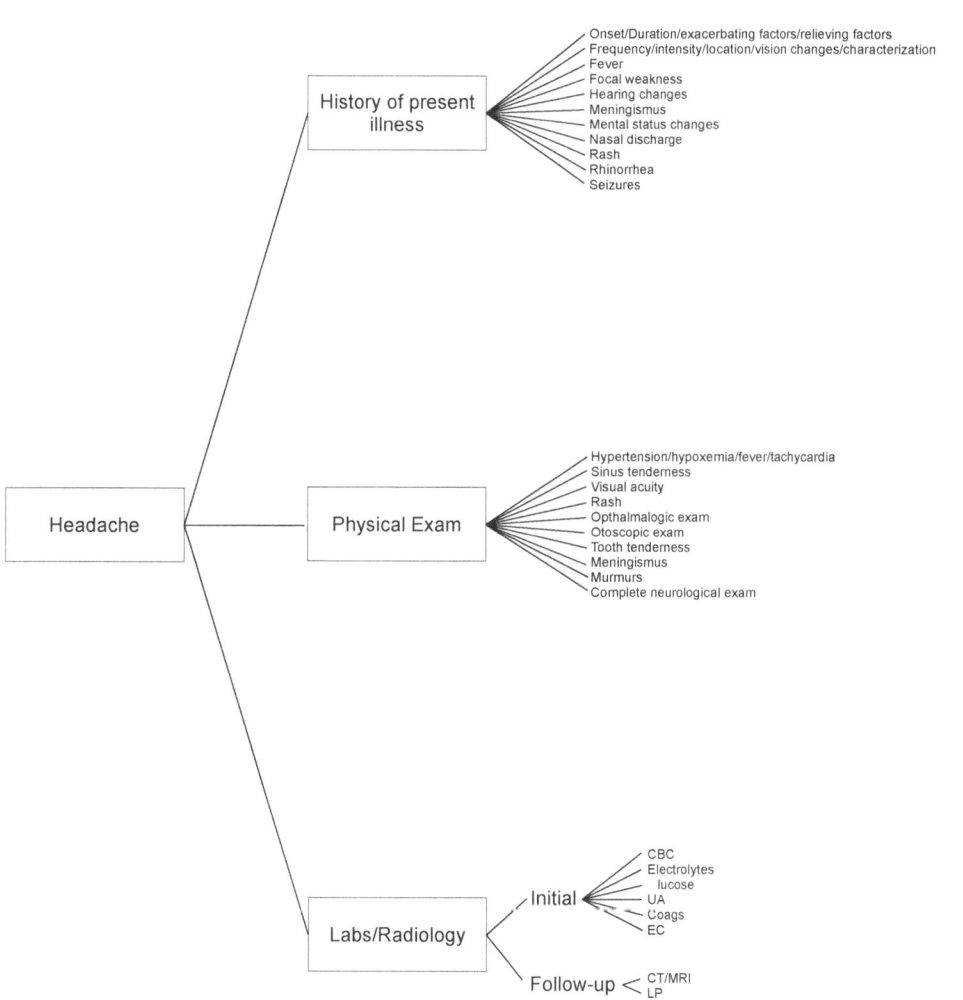

History of present illness
- Onset/Duration/exacerbating factors/relieving factors
- Frequency/intensity/location/vision changes/characterization
- Fever
- Focal weakness
- Hearing changes
- Meningismus
- Mental status changes
- Nasal discharge
- Rash
- Rhinorrhea
- Seizures

Physical Exam
- Hypertension/hypoxemia/fever/tachycardia
- Sinus tenderness
- Visual acuity
- Rash
- Opthalmalogic exam
- Otoscopic exam
- Tooth tenderness
- Meningismus
- Murmurs
- Complete neurological exam

Labs/Radiology

Initial
- CBC
- Electrolytes
- lucose
- UA
- Coags
- EC

Follow-up
- CT/MRI
- LP

# Hemoptysis

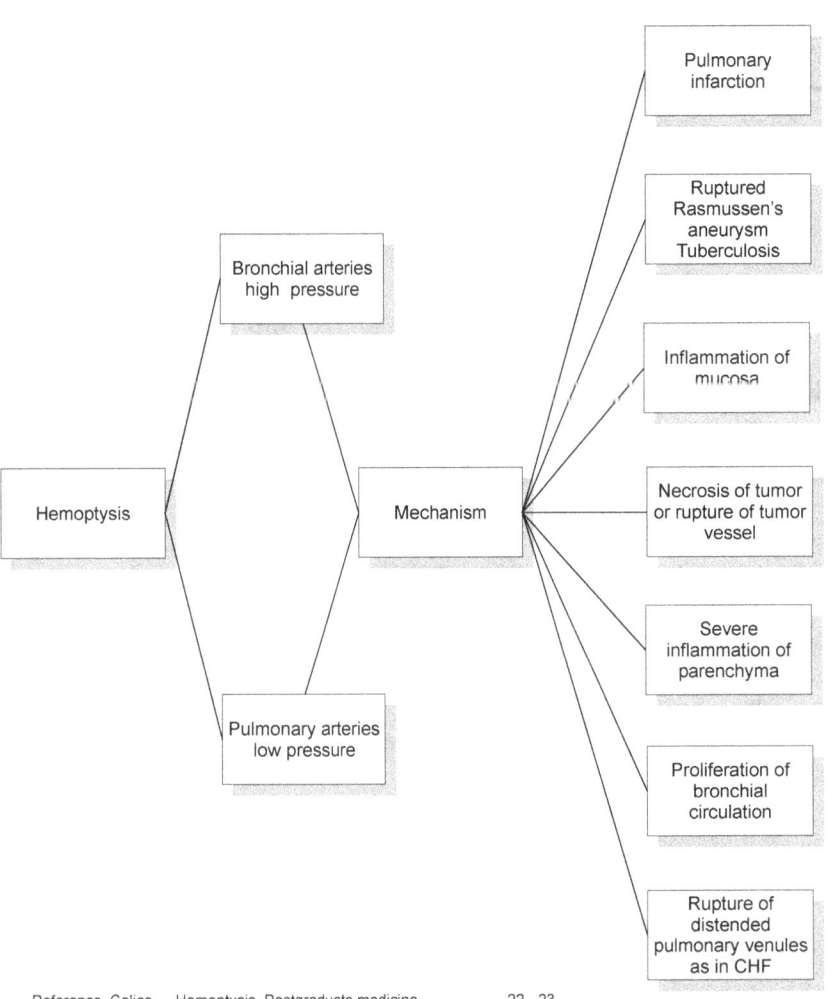

# Hemoptysis

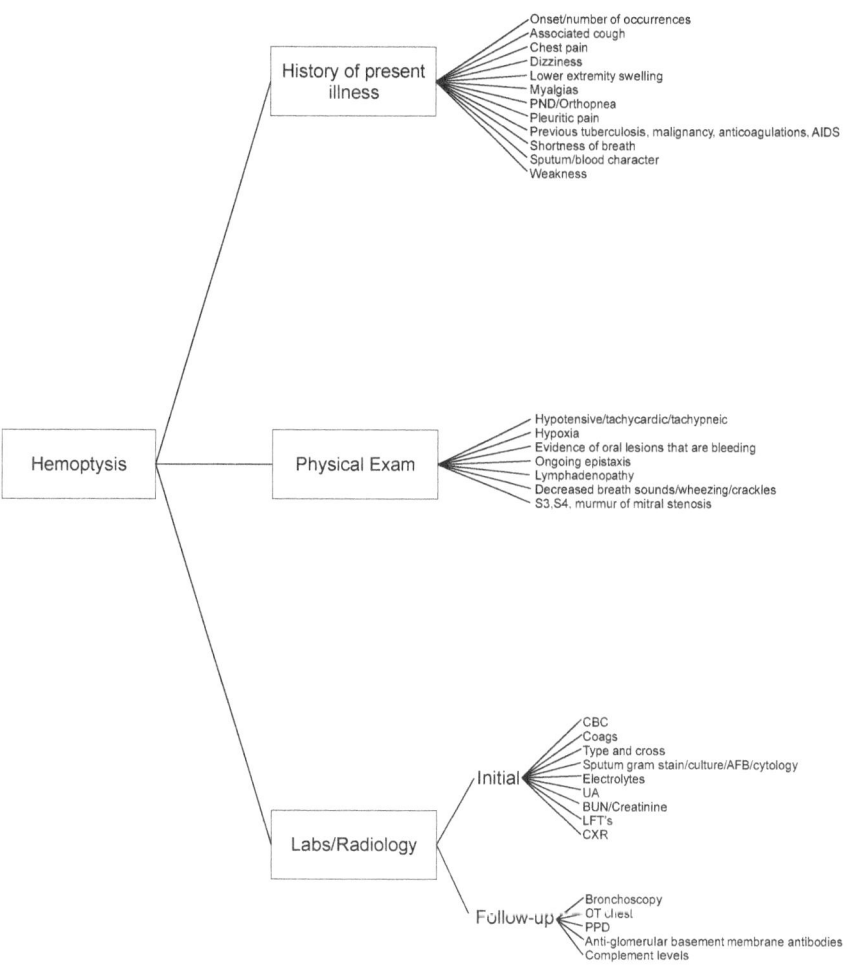

Hemoptysis

History of present illness
- Onset/number of occurrences
- Associated cough
- Chest pain
- Dizziness
- Lower extremity swelling
- Myalgias
- PND/Orthopnea
- Pleuritic pain
- Previous tuberculosis, malignancy, anticoagulations, AIDS
- Shortness of breath
- Sputum/blood character
- Weakness

Physical Exam
- Hypotensive/tachycardic/tachypneic
- Hypoxia
- Evidence of oral lesions that are bleeding
- Ongoing epistaxis
- Lymphadenopathy
- Decreased breath sounds/wheezing/crackles
- S3,S4, murmur of mitral stenosis

Labs/Radiology

Initial
- CBC
- Coags
- Type and cross
- Sputum gram stain/culture/AFB/cytology
- Electrolytes
- UA
- BUN/Creatinine
- LFT's
- CXR

Follow-up
- Bronchoscopy
- OT chest
- PPD
- Anti-glomerular basement membrane antibodies
- Complement levels

# Hirsutism

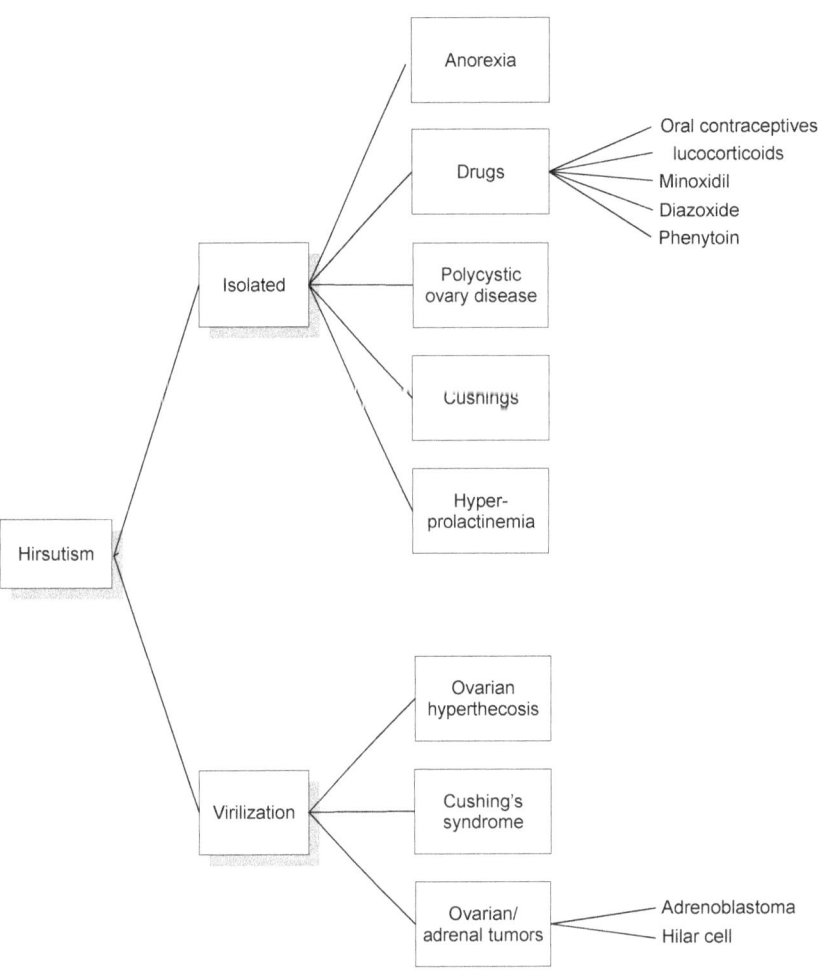

Anorexia

Drugs
— Oral contraceptives
— lucocorticoids
— Minoxidil
— Diazoxide
— Phenytoin

Isolated

Polycystic
ovary disease

Cushings

Hyper-
prolactinemia

Hirsutism

Ovarian
hyperthecosis

Cushing's
syndrome

Virilization

Ovarian/
adrenal tumors
— Adrenoblastoma
— Hilar cell

Bergfeld WF.    Hirsutism in women. Effective therapy that is safe for long-term use.    Postgrad Med. 2000 Jun;107(7):93-4, 99-10

# Hirsutism

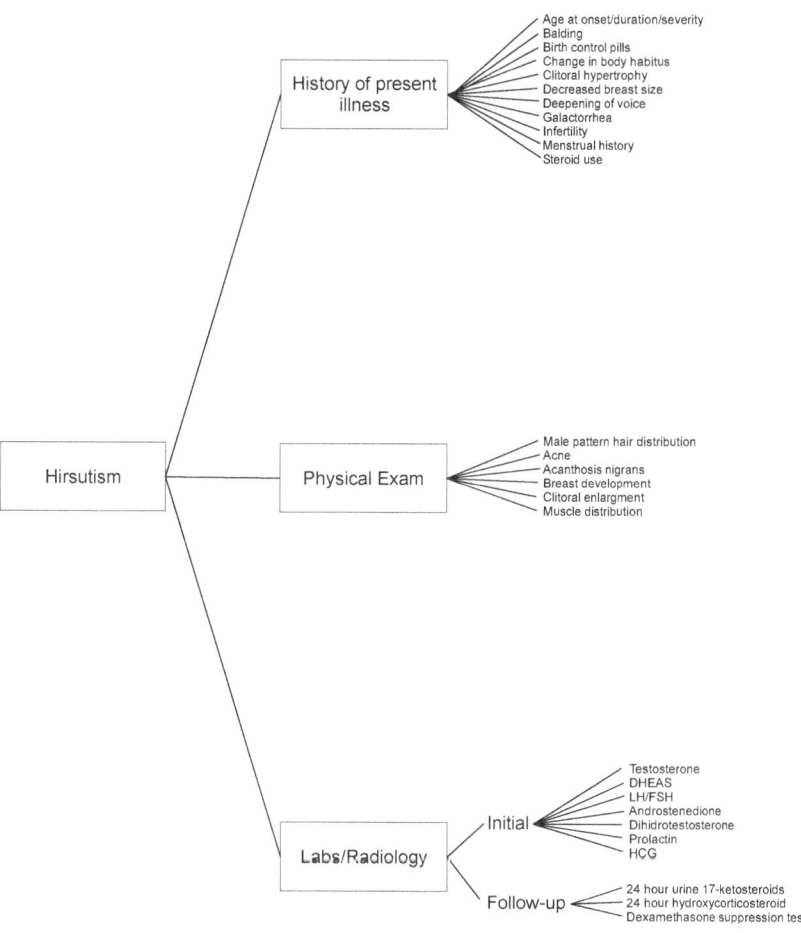

**Hirsutism**

**History of present illness**
- Age at onset/duration/severity
- Balding
- Birth control pills
- Change in body habitus
- Clitoral hypertrophy
- Decreased breast size
- Deepening of voice
- Galactorrhea
- Infertility
- Menstrual history
- Steroid use

**Physical Exam**
- Male pattern hair distribution
- Acne
- Acanthosis nigrans
- Breast development
- Clitoral enlargment
- Muscle distribution

**Labs/Radiology**

Initial
- Testosterone
- DHEAS
- LH/FSH
- Androstenedione
- Dihidrotestosterone
- Prolactin
- HCG

Follow-up
- 24 hour urine 17-ketosteroids
- 24 hour hydroxycorticosteroid
- Dexamethasone suppression test

# Hypercoagulable Patient

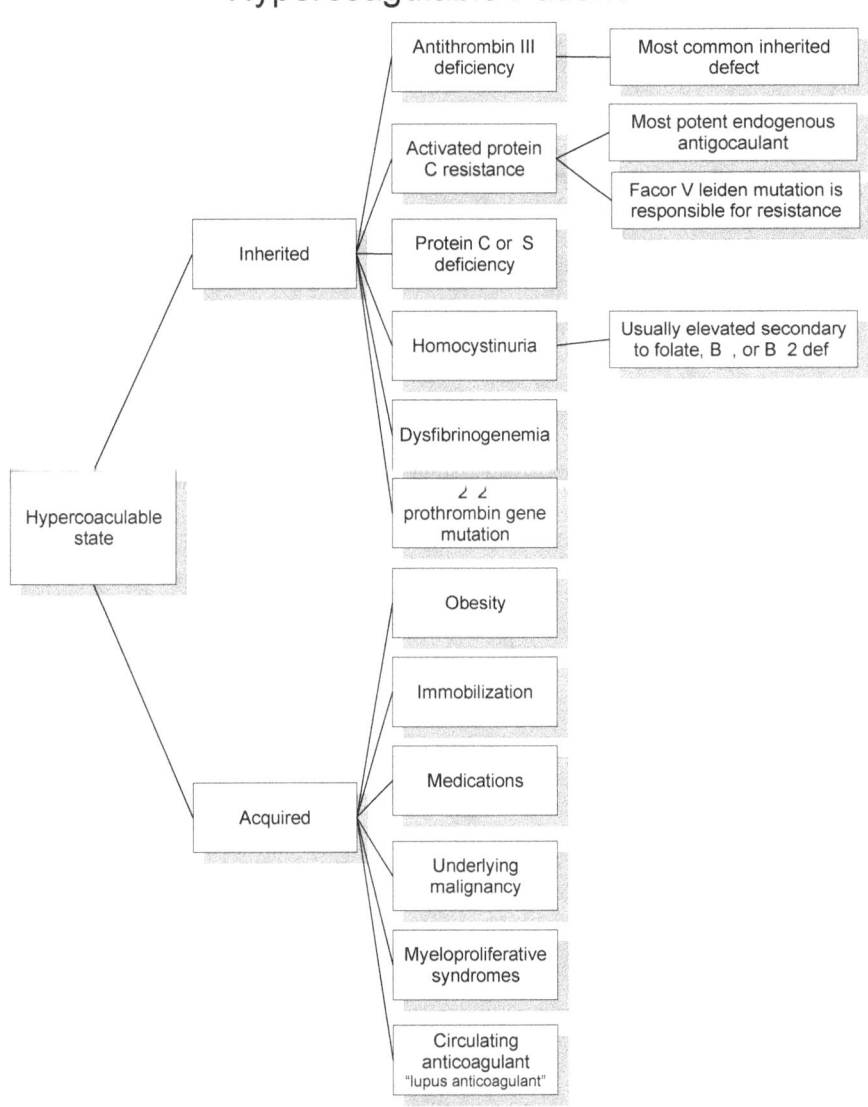

- **Hypercoaculable state**
  - **Inherited**
    - Antithrombin III deficiency → Most common inherited defect
    - Activated protein C resistance → Most potent endogenous antigocaulant
    - Activated protein C resistance → Facor V leiden mutation is responsible for resistance
    - Protein C or S deficiency
    - Homocystinuria → Usually elevated secondary to folate, B , or B 2 def
    - Dysfibrinogenemia
    - 2 2 prothrombin gene mutation
  - **Acquired**
    - Obesity
    - Immobilization
    - Medications
    - Underlying malignancy
    - Myeloproliferative syndromes
    - Circulating anticoagulant "lupus anticoagulant"

Whiteman T, et al Hypercoagulable states  Hematol Oncol Clin North Am 2    Apr  4 2 3   -

# Hypercoagulable State

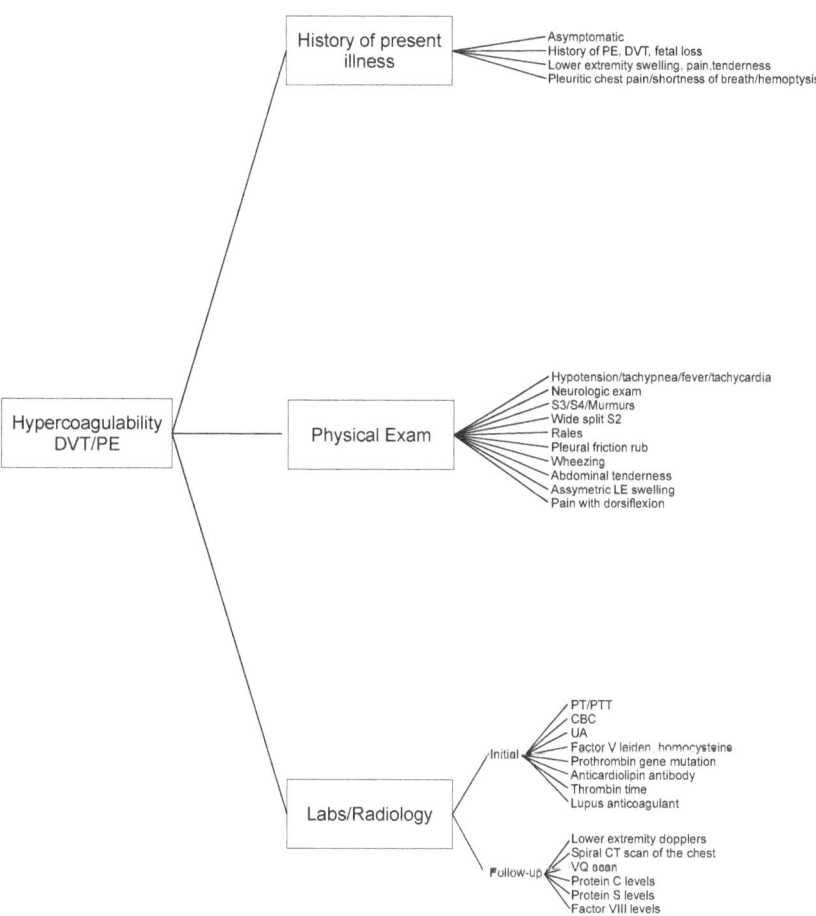

**Hypercoagulability DVT/PE**

**History of present illness**
- Asymptomatic
- History of PE, DVT, fetal loss
- Lower extremity swelling, pain, tenderness
- Pleuritic chest pain/shortness of breath/hemoptysis

**Physical Exam**
- Hypotension/tachypnea/fever/tachycardia
- Neurologic exam
- S3/S4/Murmurs
- Wide split S2
- Rales
- Pleural friction rub
- Wheezing
- Abdominal tenderness
- Assymetric LE swelling
- Pain with dorsiflexion

**Labs/Radiology**

Initial
- PT/PTT
- CBC
- UA
- Factor V leiden, homocysteine
- Prothrombin gene mutation
- Anticardiolipin antibody
- Thrombin time
- Lupus anticoagulant

Follow-up
- Lower extremity dopplers
- Spiral CT scan of the chest
- VQ scan
- Protein C levels
- Protein S levels
- Factor VIII levels

# Hyperkalemia

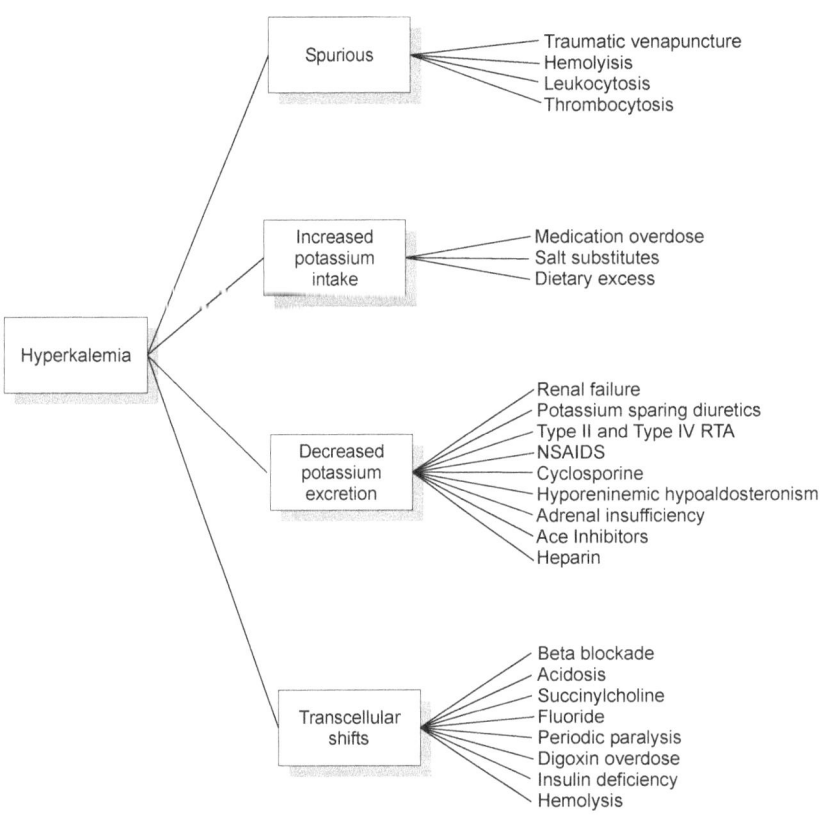

Halperin ML, et al  Potassium  Lancet      Jul    3 2    22    3 -4

# Diarrhea (Chronic)

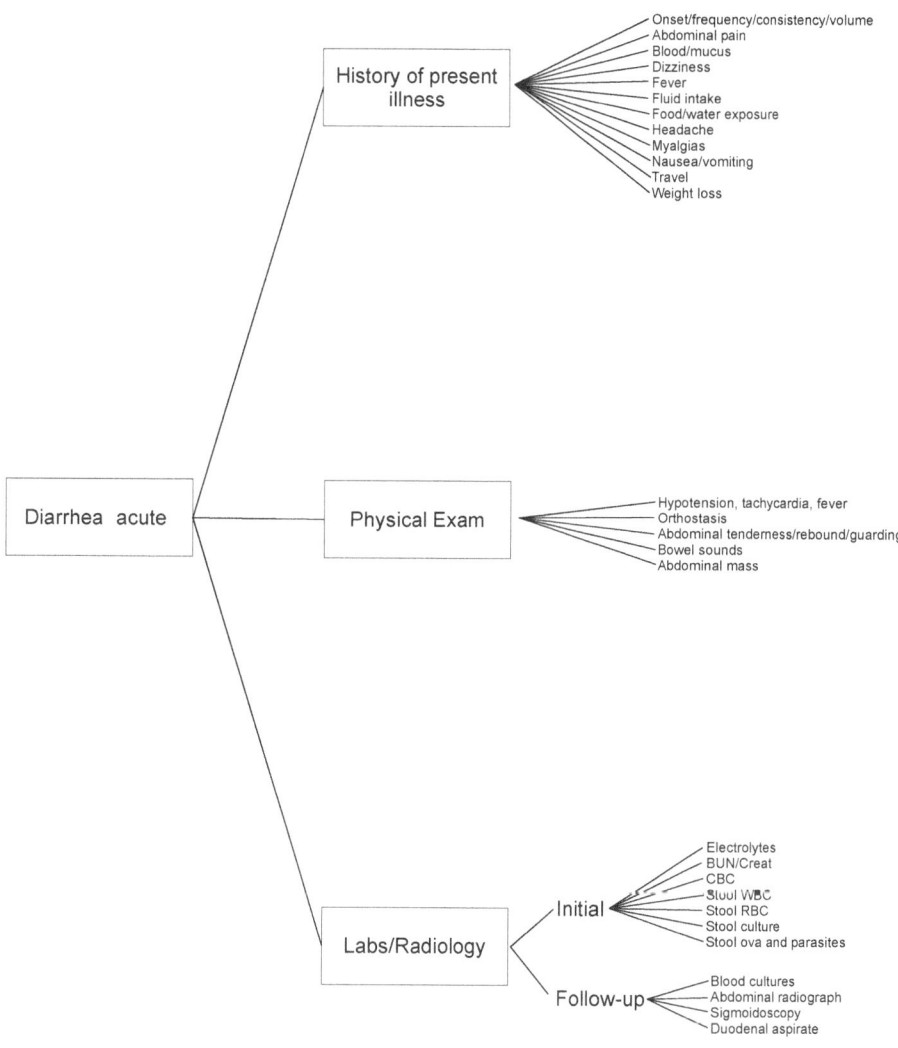

**Diarrhea acute**

**History of present illness**
- Onset/frequency/consistency/volume
- Abdominal pain
- Blood/mucus
- Dizziness
- Fever
- Fluid intake
- Food/water exposure
- Headache
- Myalgias
- Nausea/vomiting
- Travel
- Weight loss

**Physical Exam**
- Hypotension, tachycardia, fever
- Orthostasis
- Abdominal tenderness/rebound/guarding
- Bowel sounds
- Abdominal mass

**Labs/Radiology**

*Initial*
- Electrolytes
- BUN/Creat
- CBC
- Stool WBC
- Stool RBC
- Stool culture
- Stool ova and parasites

*Follow-up*
- Blood cultures
- Abdominal radiograph
- Sigmoidoscopy
- Duodenal aspirate

# Infectious Diarrhea

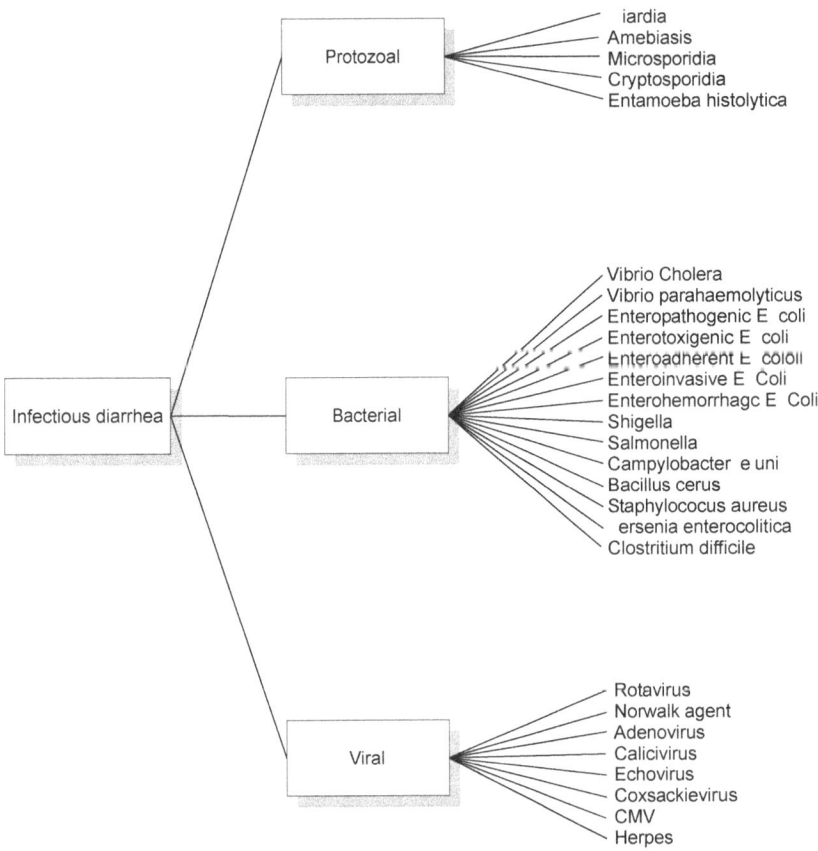

Protozoal
- iardia
- Amebiasis
- Microsporidia
- Cryptosporidia
- Entamoeba histolytica

Infectious diarrhea

Bacterial
- Vibrio Cholera
- Vibrio parahaemolyticus
- Enteropathogenic E coli
- Enterotoxigenic E coli
- Enteroadherent E coloii
- Enteroinvasive E Coli
- Enterohemorrhagc E Coli
- Shigella
- Salmonella
- Campylobacter e uni
- Bacillus cerus
- Staphylococus aureus
- ersenia enterocolitica
- Clostritium difficile

Viral
- Rotavirus
- Norwalk agent
- Adenovirus
- Calicivirus
- Echovirus
- Coxsackievirus
- CMV
- Herpes

Reference:Sutjita M, Dupont H. Guidelines on acute infectious diarrhea in adults: the practice parameters committee of the american college of gastroenterology.1997;92:1962-1975
Andreili T, Bennett J, Carpenter C, Plum F, Smith L, Cecil Essentials of Medicine. ed 3, Philadelphia, 1993, W.B. Saunders Company. page 67

# Dizziness

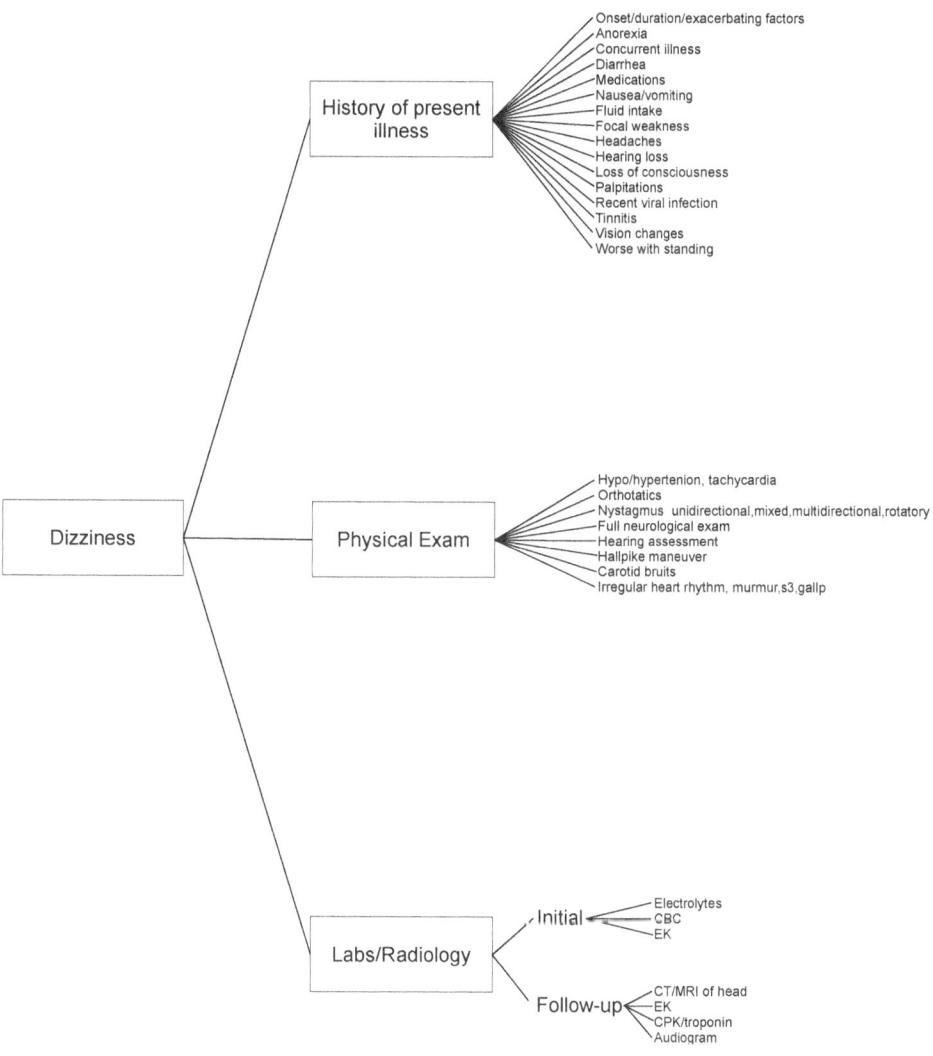

**History of present illness**
- Onset/duration/exacerbating factors
- Anorexia
- Concurrent illness
- Diarrhea
- Medications
- Nausea/vomiting
- Fluid intake
- Focal weakness
- Headaches
- Hearing loss
- Loss of consciousness
- Palpitations
- Recent viral infection
- Tinnitis
- Vision changes
- Worse with standing

**Physical Exam**
- Hypo/hypertenion, tachycardia
- Orthotatics
- Nystagmus  unidirectional,mixed,multidirectional,rotatory
- Full neurological exam
- Hearing assessment
- Hallpike maneuver
- Carotid bruits
- Irregular heart rhythm, murmur,s3,gallp

**Labs/Radiology**

Initial
- Electrolytes
- CBC
- EK

Follow-up
- CT/MRI of head
- EK
- CPK/troponin
- Audiogram

# Dizziness

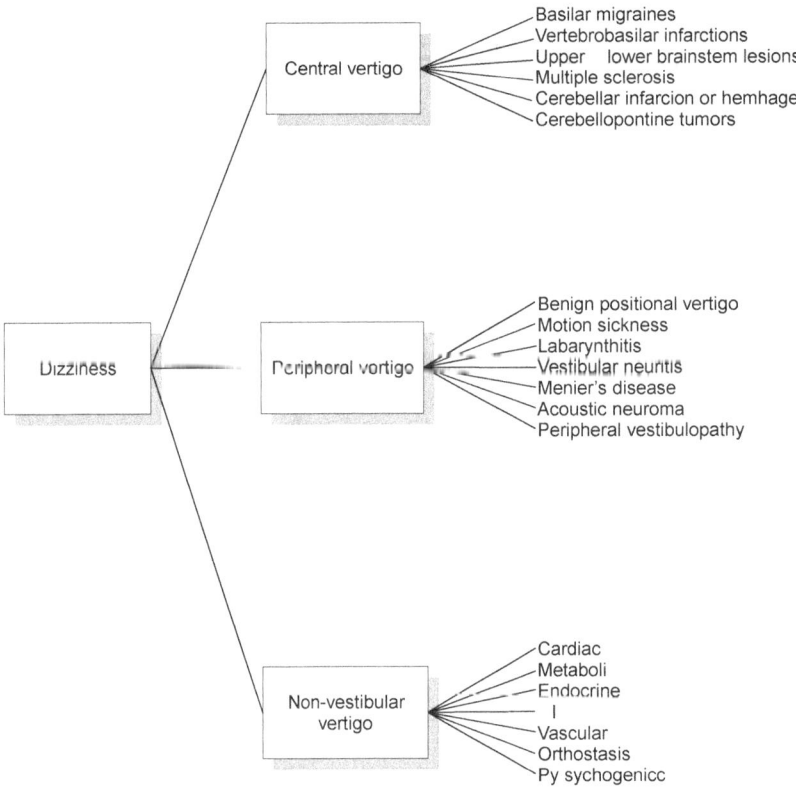

**Dizziness**

**Central vertigo**
- Basilar migraines
- Vertebrobasilar infarctions
- Upper    lower brainstem lesions
- Multiple sclerosis
- Cerebellar infarcion or hemhage
- Cerebellopontine tumors

**Peripheral vortigo**
- Benign positional vertigo
- Motion sickness
- Labarynthitis
- Vestibular neuritis
- Menier's disease
- Acoustic neuroma
- Peripheral vestibulopathy

**Non-vestibular vertigo**
- Cardiac
- Metaboli
- Endocrine
- I
- Vascular
- Orthostasis
- Py sychogenicc

Baloh R. The dizzy patient. Postgraduate Medicine;1999;105(2);161-172.
Reference: Walker J, Barnes B, Dizzyness. Emergency medicine clinics of North America, 1998;16(4);845-875

# Dysphagia

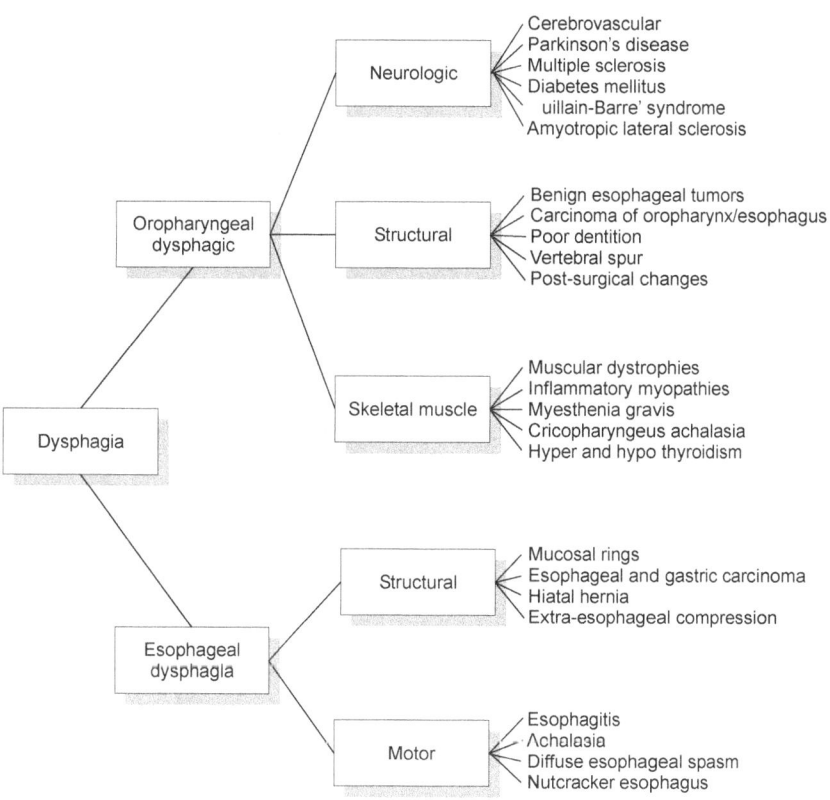

Reference: Barloon J, Bergus G, Lu C. Diagnostic imaging in the evaluation of dysphagia. American family physician1996;53:535-546.

Andreili T, Bennett J, Carpenter C, Plum F, Smith L. Cecil Essentials of Medicine, ed 3, Philadelphia, 1993, W.B. Saunders Company. page 284

# Dysphagia

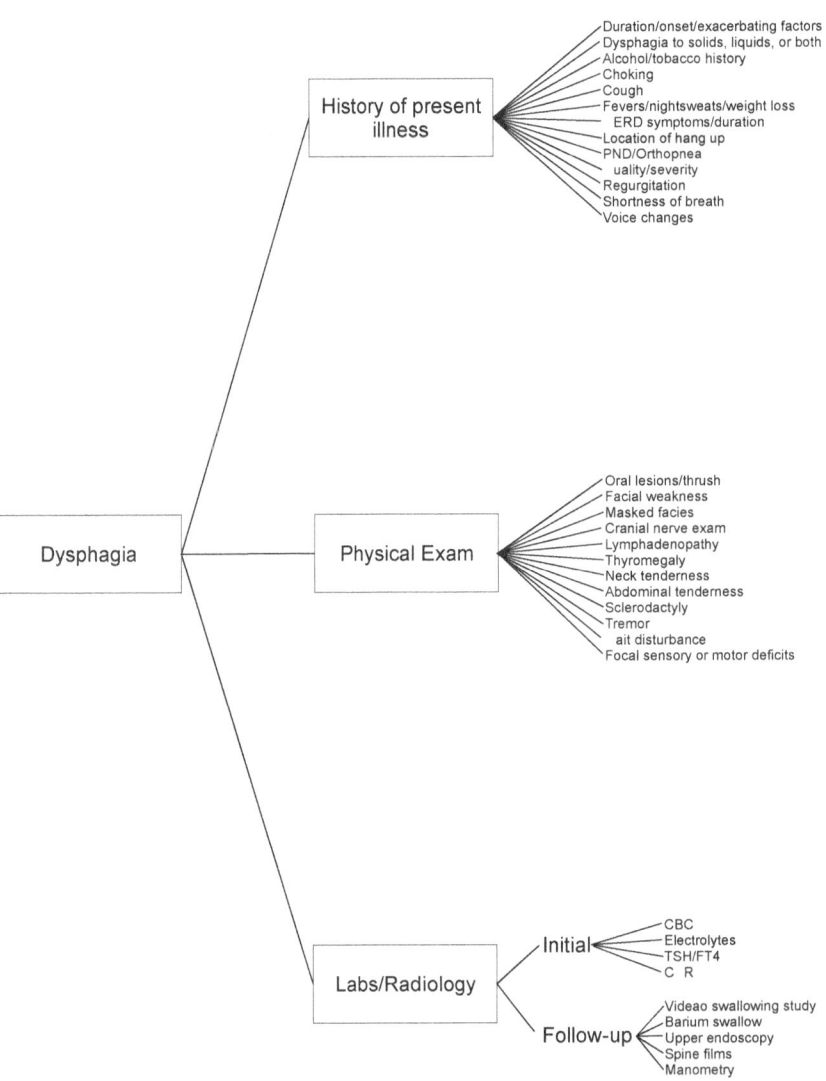

**Dysphagia**

**History of present illness**
- Duration/onset/exacerbating factors
- Dysphagia to solids, liquids, or both
- Alcohol/tobacco history
- Choking
- Cough
- Fevers/nightsweats/weight loss
- ERD symptoms/duration
- Location of hang up
- PND/Orthopnea
- uality/severity
- Regurgitation
- Shortness of breath
- Voice changes

**Physical Exam**
- Oral lesions/thrush
- Facial weakness
- Masked facies
- Cranial nerve exam
- Lymphadenopathy
- Thyromegaly
- Neck tenderness
- Abdominal tenderness
- Sclerodactyly
- Tremor
- ait disturbance
- Focal sensory or motor deficits

**Labs/Radiology**

Initial
- CBC
- Electrolytes
- TSH/FT4
- C R

Follow-up
- Videao swallowing study
- Barium swallow
- Upper endoscopy
- Spine films
- Manometry

# Dyspnea  Acute

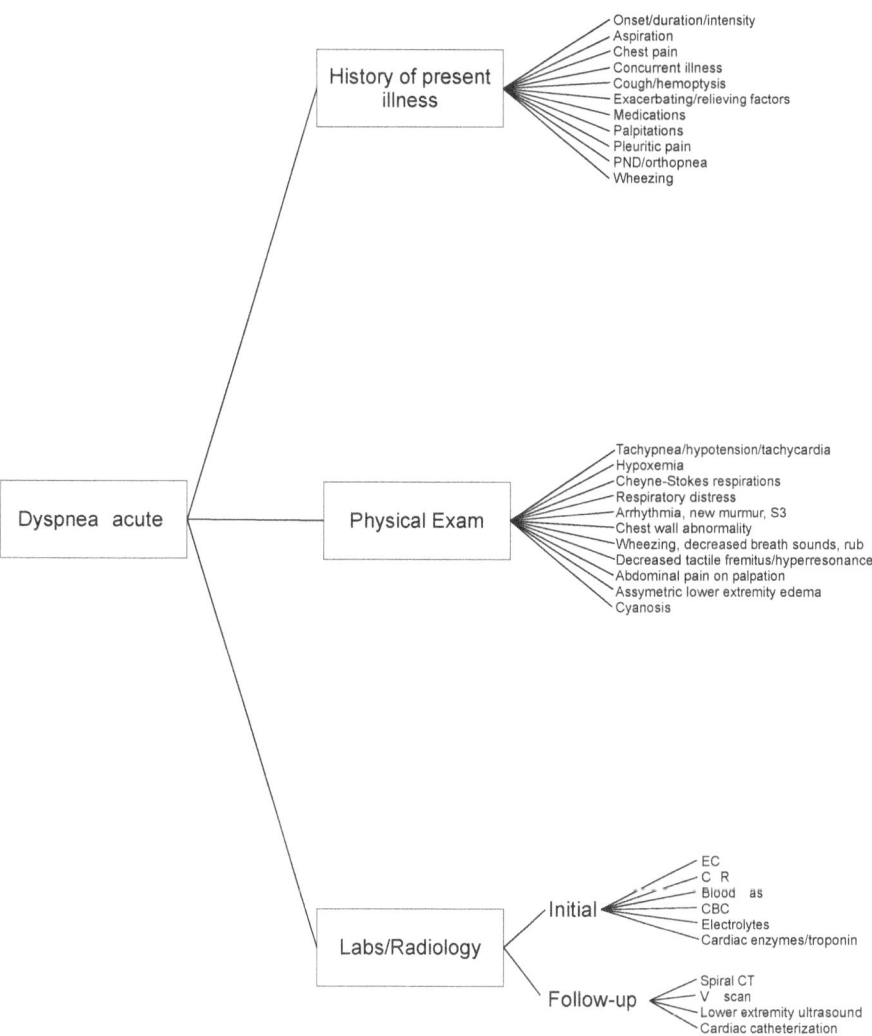

History of present illness
- Onset/duration/intensity
- Aspiration
- Chest pain
- Concurrent illness
- Cough/hemoptysis
- Exacerbating/relieving factors
- Medications
- Palpitations
- Pleuritic pain
- PND/orthopnea
- Wheezing

Dyspnea  acute

Physical Exam
- Tachypnea/hypotension/tachycardia
- Hypoxemia
- Cheyne-Stokes respirations
- Respiratory distress
- Arrhythmia, new murmur, S3
- Chest wall abnormality
- Wheezing, decreased breath sounds, rub
- Decreased tactile fremitus/hyperresonance
- Abdominal pain on palpation
- Assymetric lower extremity edema
- Cyanosis

Labs/Radiology

Initial
- EC
- C  R
- Blood  as
- CBC
- Electrolytes
- Cardiac enzymes/troponin

Follow-up
- Spiral CT
- V    scan
- Lower extremity ultrasound
- Cardiac catheterization

# Acute Dyspnea

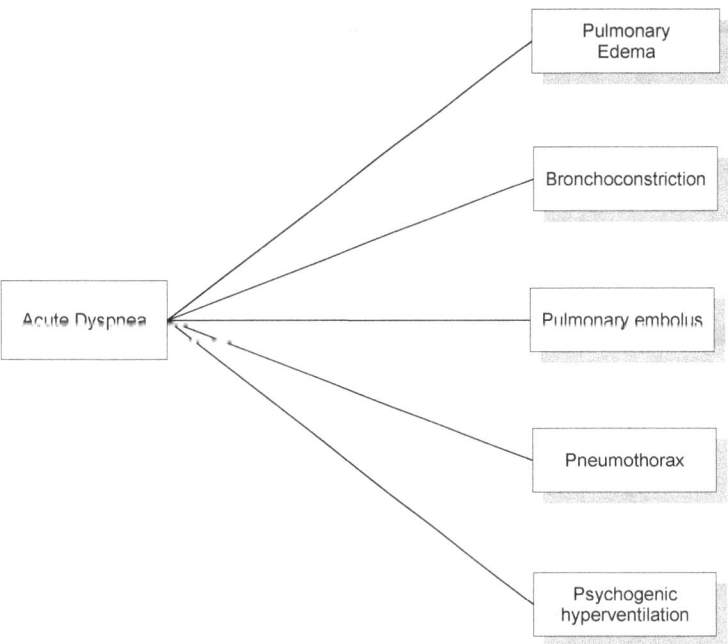

Acute Dyspnea

- Pulmonary Edema
- Bronchoconstriction
- Pulmonary embolus
- Pneumothorax
- Psychogenic hyperventilation

Weisman I, Zeballos R. Clinical evaluation of unexplained dyspnea. Cardiologia 1996;41(7):621-34.

# Eosinophilia

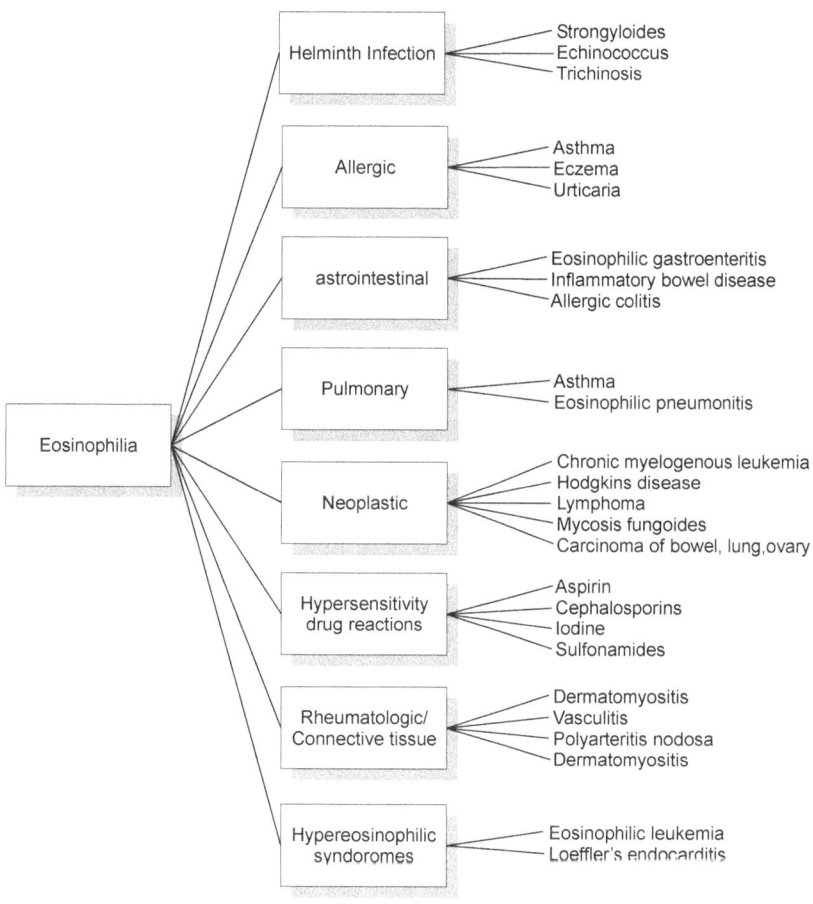

Reference: Bain B. Hypereosinophilia. Curr Opin Hematol 2000;7(1):21-5.

# Eosinophilia

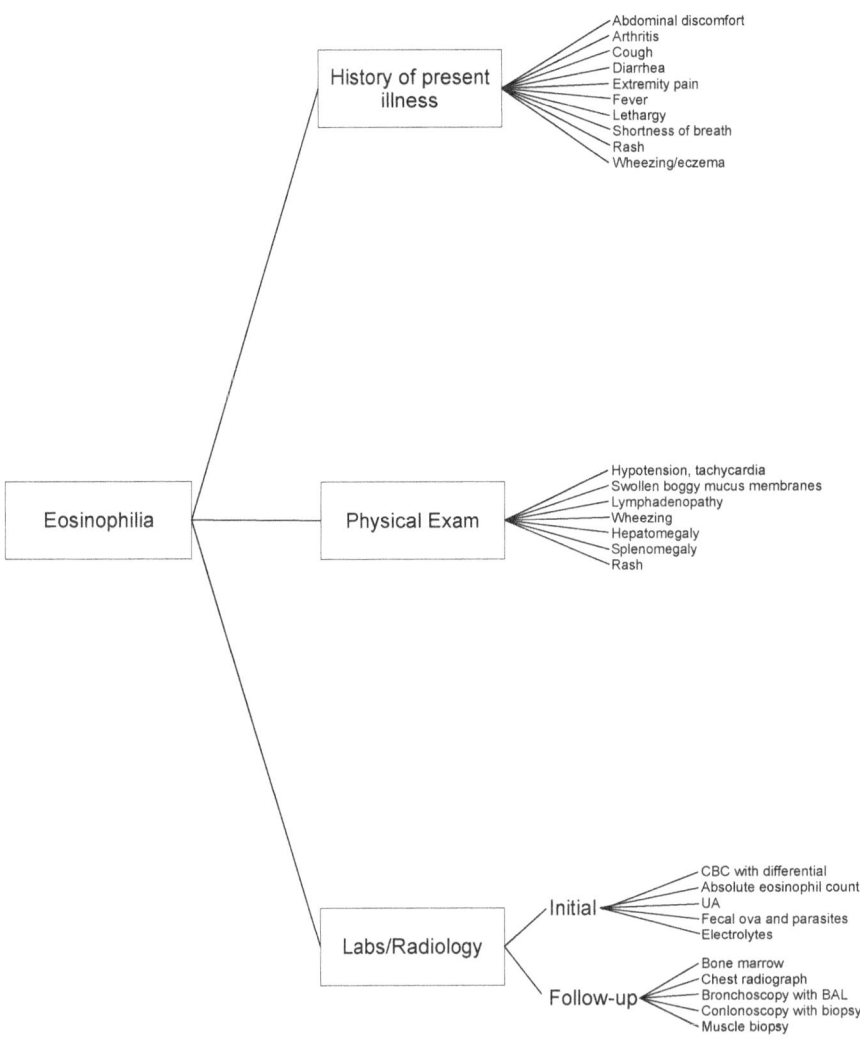

**History of present illness**
- Abdominal discomfort
- Arthritis
- Cough
- Diarrhea
- Extremity pain
- Fever
- Lethargy
- Shortness of breath
- Rash
- Wheezing/eczema

**Physical Exam**
- Hypotension, tachycardia
- Swollen boggy mucus membranes
- Lymphadenopathy
- Wheezing
- Hepatomegaly
- Splenomegaly
- Rash

**Labs/Radiology**

Initial
- CBC with differential
- Absolute eosinophil count
- UA
- Fecal ova and parasites
- Electrolytes

Follow-up
- Bone marrow
- Chest radiograph
- Bronchoscopy with BAL
- Conlonoscopy with biopsy
- Muscle biopsy

www.flash-med.com

# alactorrhea

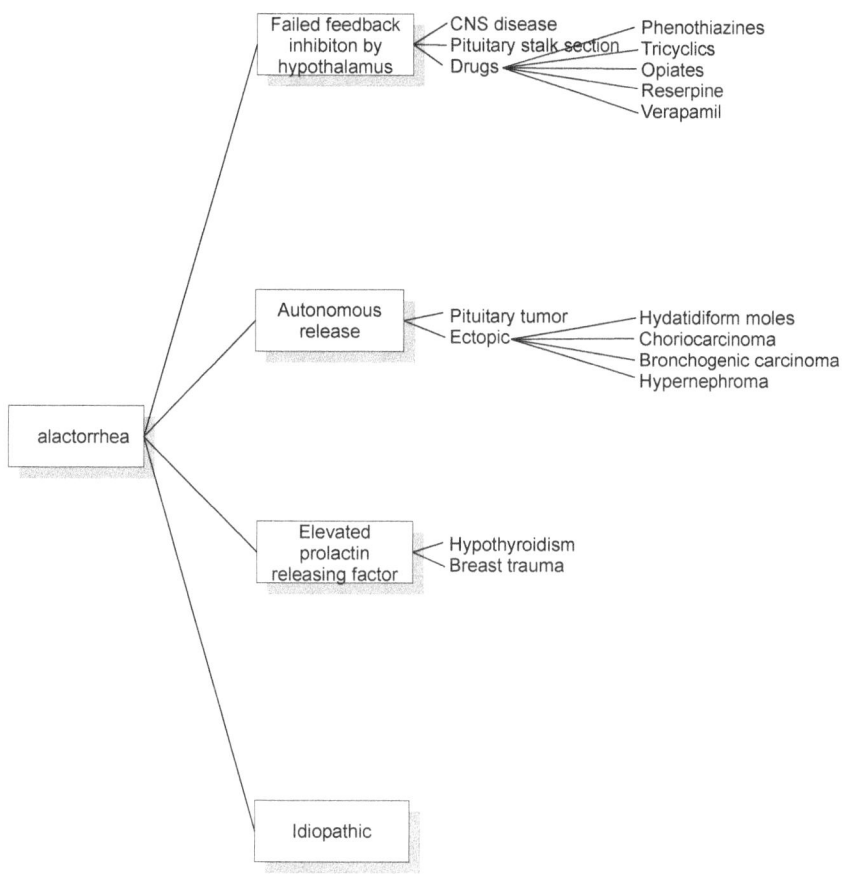

Reference: Haney A. Galactorrhea. Curr Ther Endocrinol Metab 1997;6:393-6.

# Galactorrhea

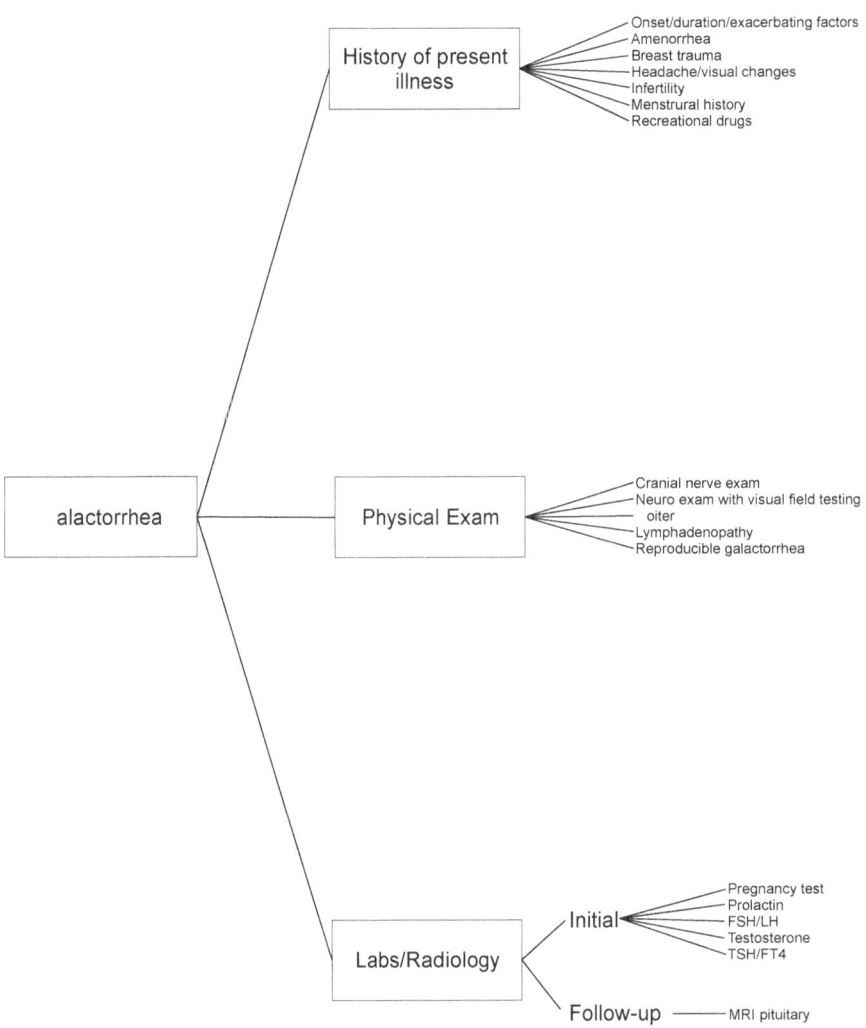

**History of present illness**
- Onset/duration/exacerbating factors
- Amenorrhea
- Breast trauma
- Headache/visual changes
- Infertility
- Menstrural history
- Recreational drugs

**alactorrhea**

**Physical Exam**
- Cranial nerve exam
- Neuro exam with visual field testing
- oiter
- Lymphadenopathy
- Reproducible galactorrhea

**Labs/Radiology**

Initial
- Pregnancy test
- Prolactin
- FSH/LH
- Testosterone
- TSH/FT4

Follow-up — MRI pituitary

# ynecomastia

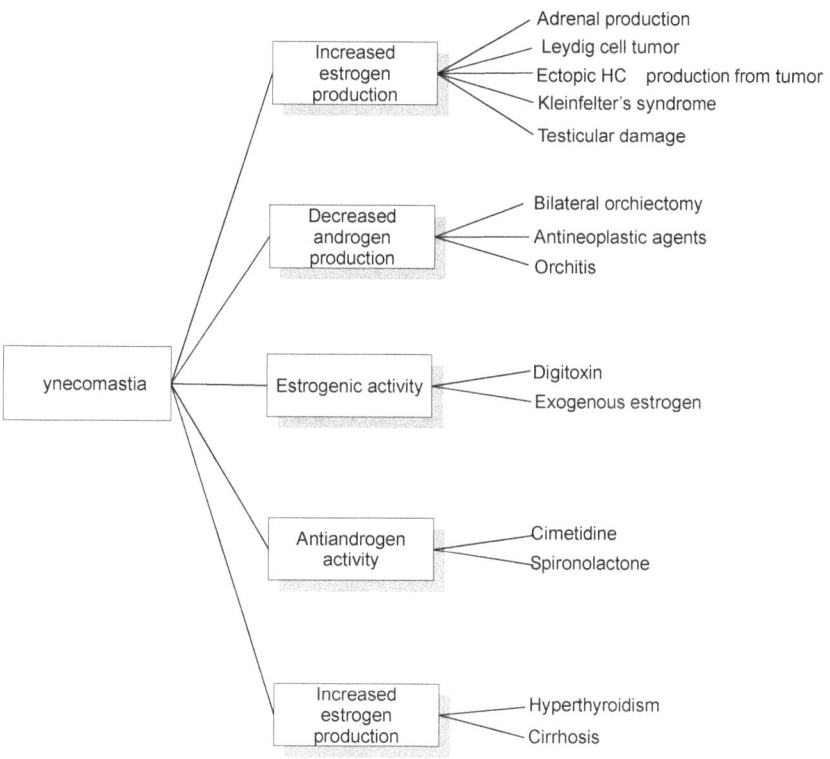

Increased estrogen production
- Adrenal production
- Leydig cell tumor
- Ectopic HC    production from tumor
- Kleinfelter's syndrome
- Testicular damage

Decreased androgen production
- Bilateral orchiectomy
- Antineoplastic agents
- Orchitis

Estrogenic activity
- Digitoxin
- Exogenous estrogen

Antiandrogen activity
- Cimetidine
- Spironolactone

Increased estrogen production
- Hyperthyroidism
- Cirrhosis

Neuman J. Evaluation and treatement of gynecomastia. Am Fam Physician 1997;55(5):1835-44,1849-50.

www.flash-med.com

# Gynecomastia

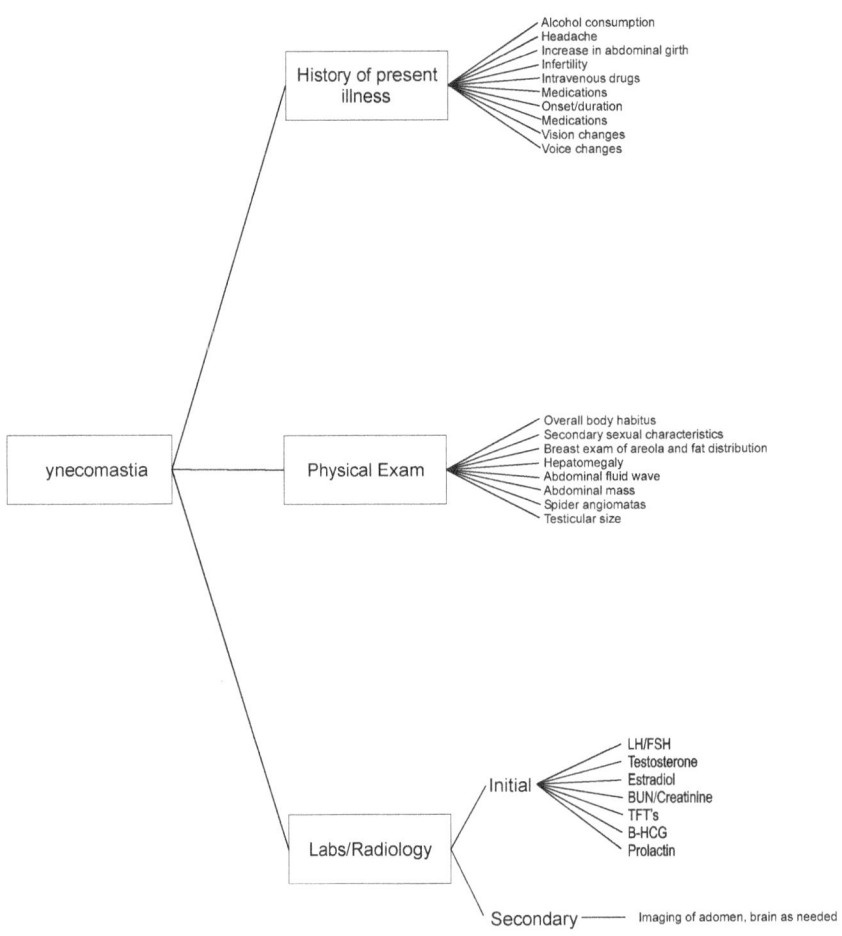

# Headache

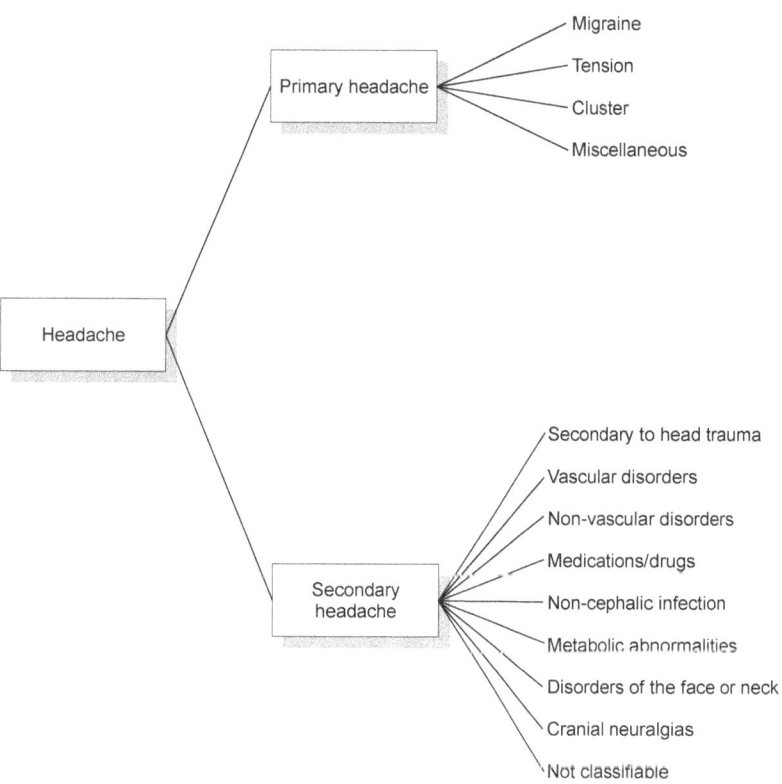

Primary headache
- Migraine
- Tension
- Cluster
- Miscellaneous

Secondary headache
- Secondary to head trauma
- Vascular disorders
- Non-vascular disorders
- Medications/drugs
- Non-cephalic infection
- Metabolic abnormalities
- Disorders of the face or neck
- Cranial neuralgias
- Not classifiable

Lipton RB Classification and epidemiology of headache - Clin Cornerstone -                  -

# Headache

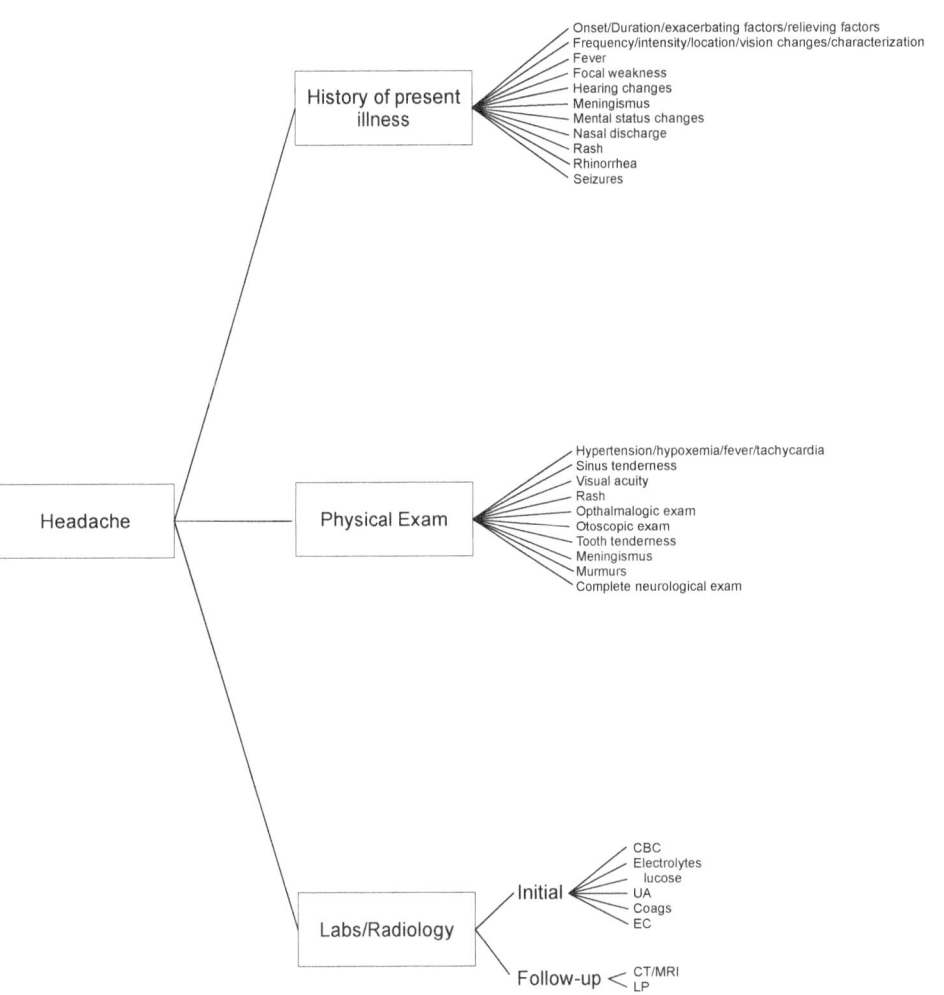

**History of present illness**
- Onset/Duration/exacerbating factors/relieving factors
- Frequency/intensity/location/vision changes/characterization
- Fever
- Focal weakness
- Hearing changes
- Meningismus
- Mental status changes
- Nasal discharge
- Rash
- Rhinorrhea
- Seizures

**Physical Exam**
- Hypertension/hypoxemia/fever/tachycardia
- Sinus tenderness
- Visual acuity
- Rash
- Opthalmalogic exam
- Otoscopic exam
- Tooth tenderness
- Meningismus
- Murmurs
- Complete neurological exam

**Labs/Radiology**
- Initial
  - CBC
  - Electrolytes
  - lucose
  - UA
  - Coags
  - EC
- Follow-up
  - CT/MRI
  - LP

# Hemoptysis

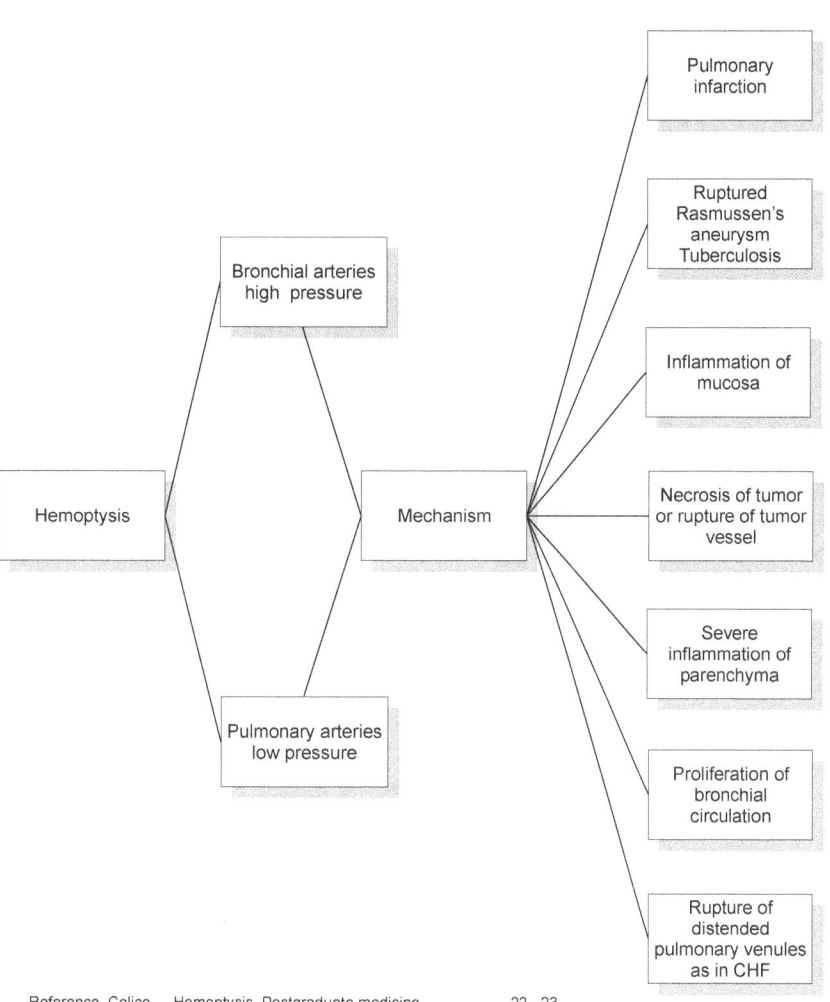

# Hemoptysis

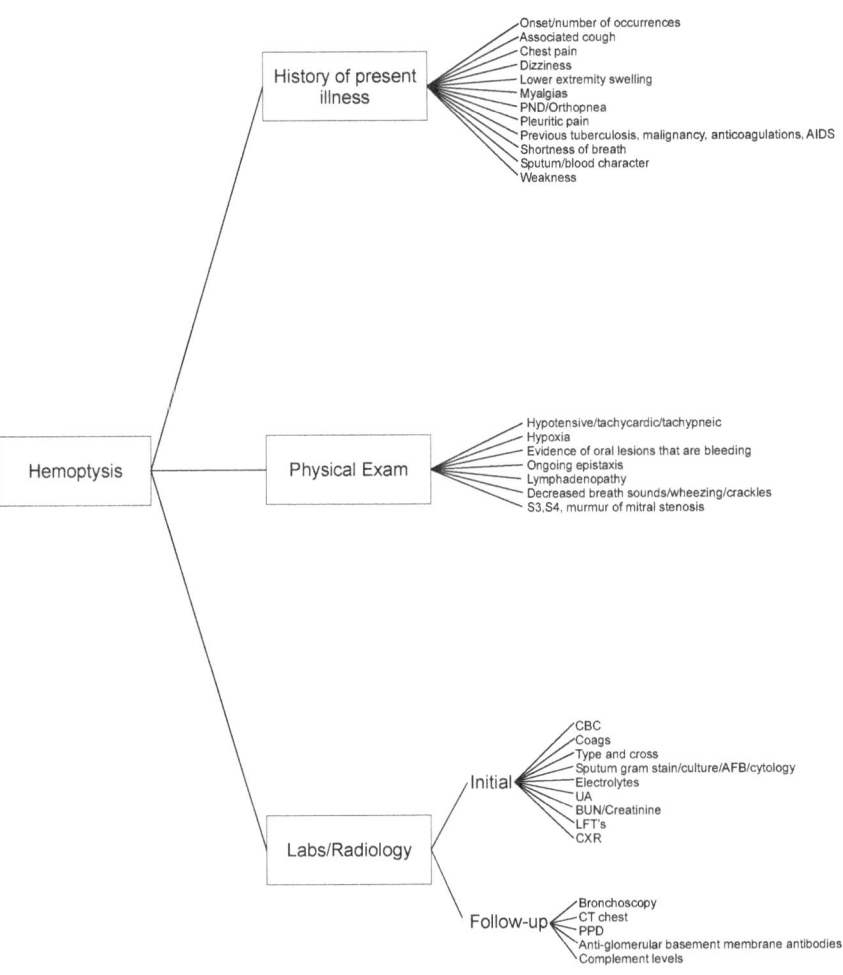

**History of present illness**
- Onset/number of occurrences
- Associated cough
- Chest pain
- Dizziness
- Lower extremity swelling
- Myalgias
- PND/Orthopnea
- Pleuritic pain
- Previous tuberculosis, malignancy, anticoagulations, AIDS
- Shortness of breath
- Sputum/blood character
- Weakness

**Physical Exam**
- Hypotensive/tachycardic/tachypneic
- Hypoxia
- Evidence of oral lesions that are bleeding
- Ongoing epistaxis
- Lymphadenopathy
- Decreased breath sounds/wheezing/crackles
- S3,S4, murmur of mitral stenosis

**Labs/Radiology**

Initial
- CBC
- Coags
- Type and cross
- Sputum gram stain/culture/AFB/cytology
- Electrolytes
- UA
- BUN/Creatinine
- LFT's
- CXR

Follow-up
- Bronchoscopy
- CT chest
- PPD
- Anti-glomerular basement membrane antibodies
- Complement levels

# Hirsutism

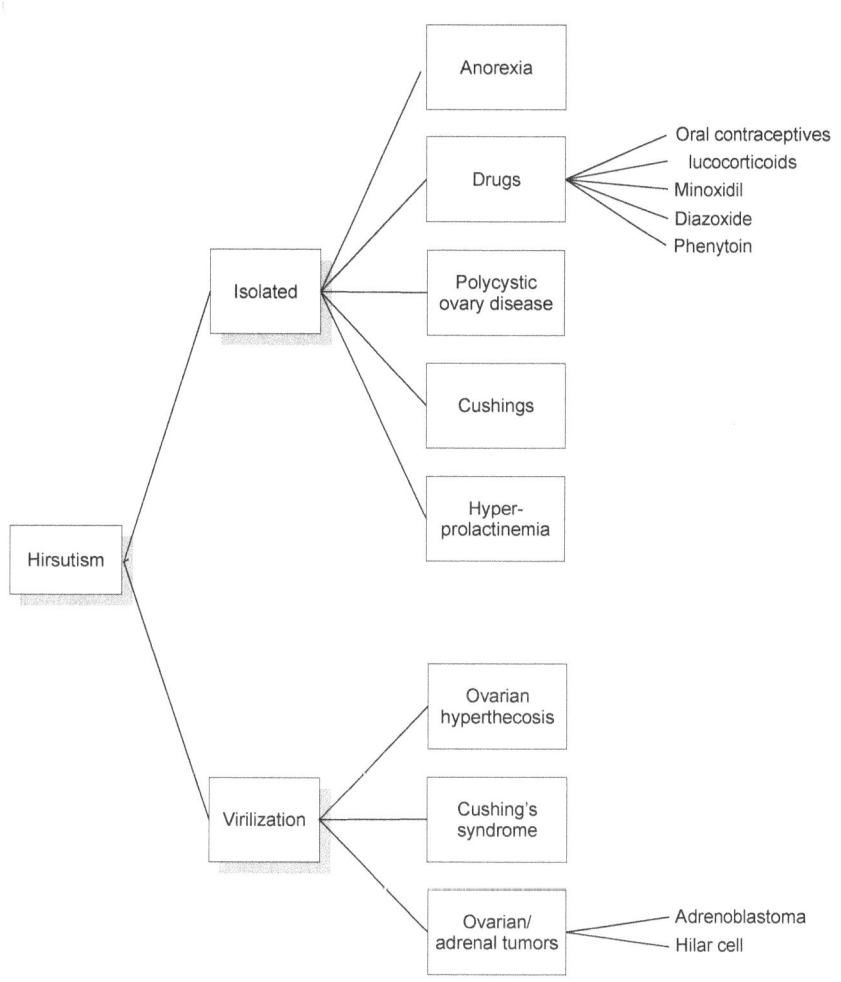

Bergfeld WF.   Hirsutism in women. Effective therapy that is safe for long-term use.   Postgrad Med. 2000 Jun;107(7):93-4, 99-104

# Hirsutism

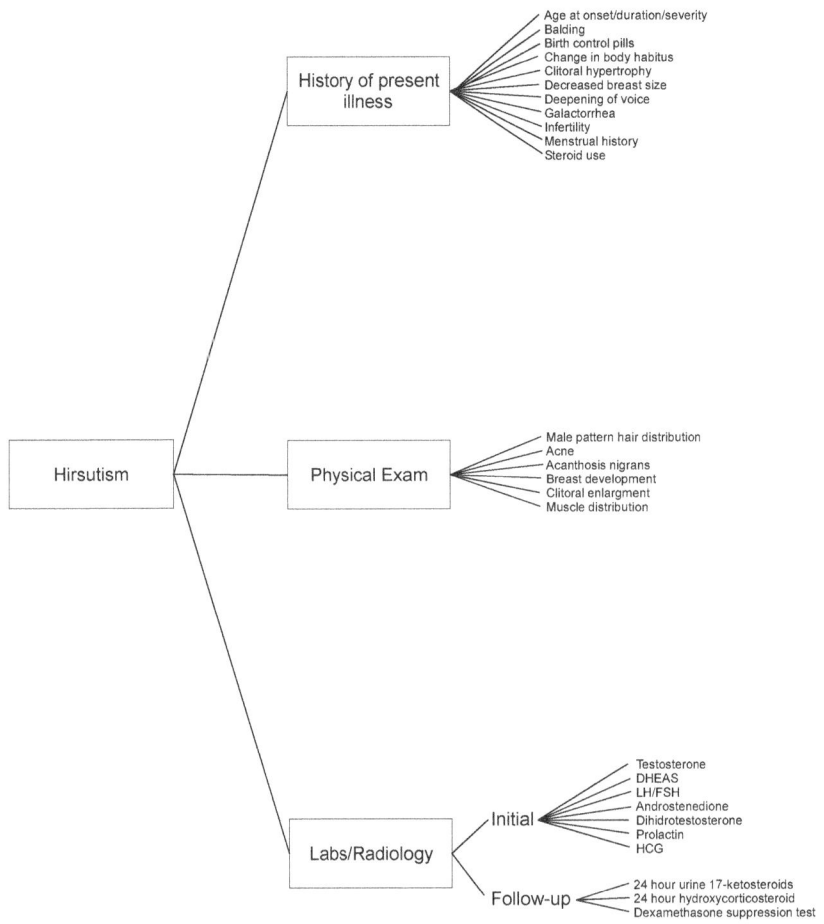

**History of present illness**
- Age at onset/duration/severity
- Balding
- Birth control pills
- Change in body habitus
- Clitoral hypertrophy
- Decreased breast size
- Deepening of voice
- Galactorrhea
- Infertility
- Menstrual history
- Steroid use

**Physical Exam**
- Male pattern hair distribution
- Acne
- Acanthosis nigrans
- Breast development
- Clitoral enlargment
- Muscle distribution

**Labs/Radiology**

Initial
- Testosterone
- DHEAS
- LH/FSH
- Androstenedione
- Dihidrotestosterone
- Prolactin
- HCG

Follow-up
- 24 hour urine 17-ketosteroids
- 24 hour hydroxycorticosteroid
- Dexamethasone suppression test

# Hypercoagulable Patient

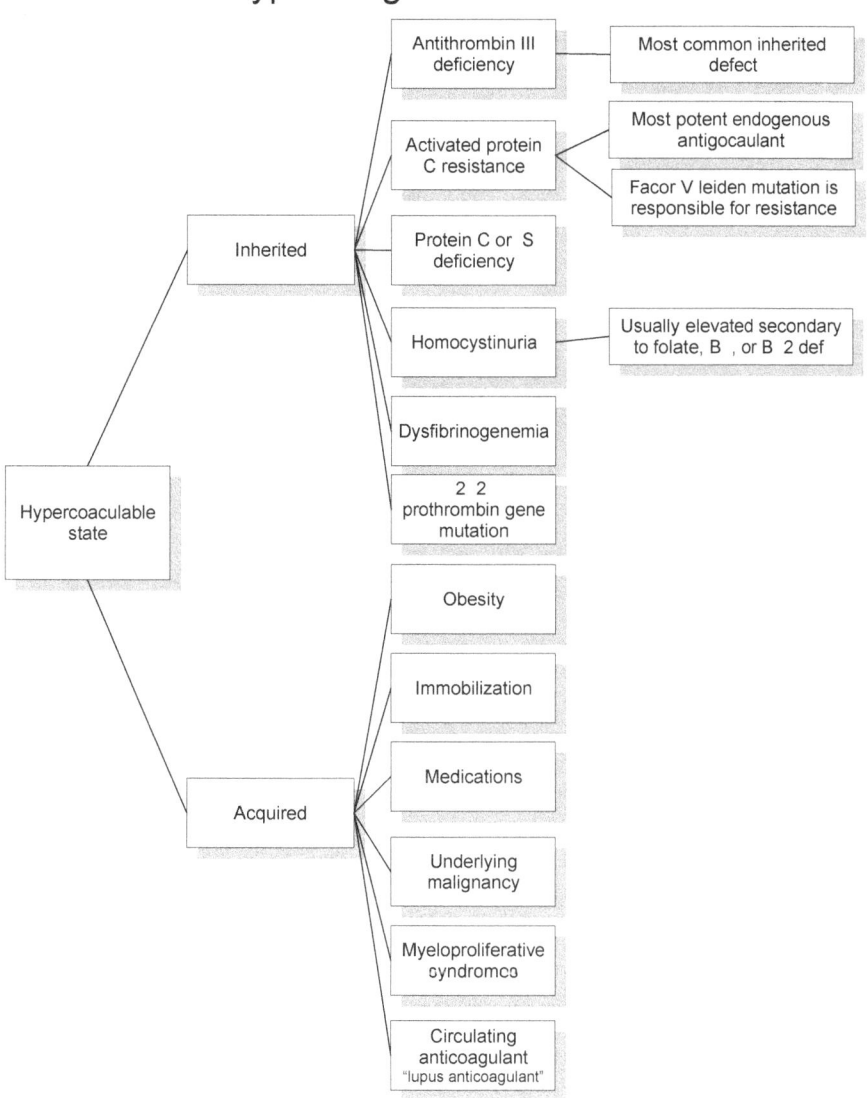

Whiteman T, et al Hypercoagulable states  Hematol Oncol Clin North Am  2    Apr  4 2 3  -   viii

# Hypercoagulable State

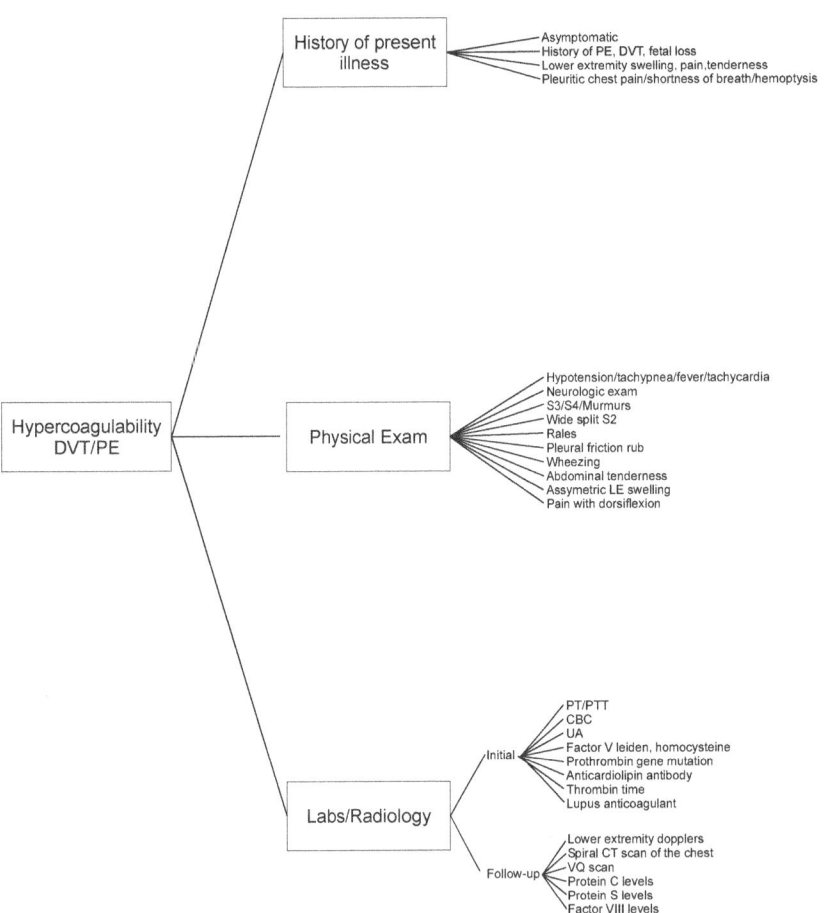

Hypercoagulability DVT/PE

**History of present illness**
- Asymptomatic
- History of PE, DVT, fetal loss
- Lower extremity swelling, pain,tenderness
- Pleuritic chest pain/shortness of breath/hemoptysis

**Physical Exam**
- Hypotension/tachypnea/fever/tachycardia
- Neurologic exam
- S3/S4/Murmurs
- Wide split S2
- Rales
- Pleural friction rub
- Wheezing
- Abdominal tenderness
- Assymetric LE swelling
- Pain with dorsiflexion

**Labs/Radiology**

Initial
- PT/PTT
- CBC
- UA
- Factor V leiden, homocysteine
- Prothrombin gene mutation
- Anticardiolipin antibody
- Thrombin time
- Lupus anticoagulant

Follow-up
- Lower extremity dopplers
- Spiral CT scan of the chest
- VQ scan
- Protein C levels
- Protein S levels
- Factor VIII levels

# Hyperkalemia

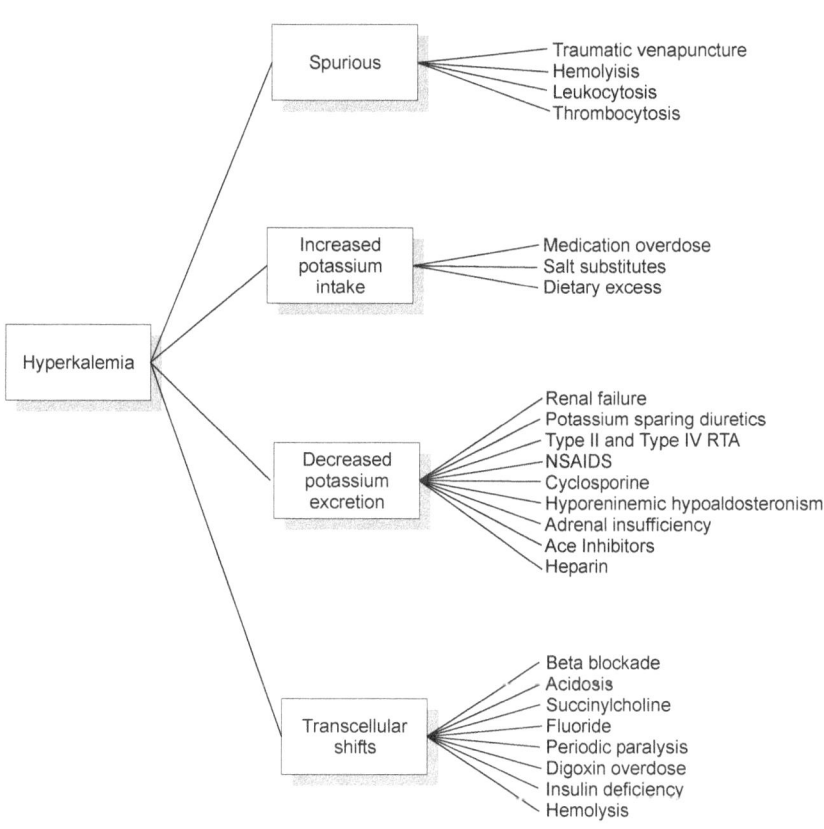

Spurious
- Traumatic venapuncture
- Hemolyisis
- Leukocytosis
- Thrombocytosis

Increased potassium intake
- Medication overdose
- Salt substitutes
- Dietary excess

Hyperkalemia

Decreased potassium excretion
- Renal failure
- Potassium sparing diuretics
- Type II and Type IV RTA
- NSAIDS
- Cyclosporine
- Hyporeninemic hypoaldosteronism
- Adrenal insufficiency
- Ace Inhibitors
- Heparin

Transcellular shifts
- Beta blockade
- Acidosis
- Succinylcholine
- Fluoride
- Periodic paralysis
- Digoxin overdose
- Insulin deficiency
- Hemolysis

Halperin ML, et al  Potassium  Lancet      Jul    3 2    22   3 -4

# Hyperkalemia

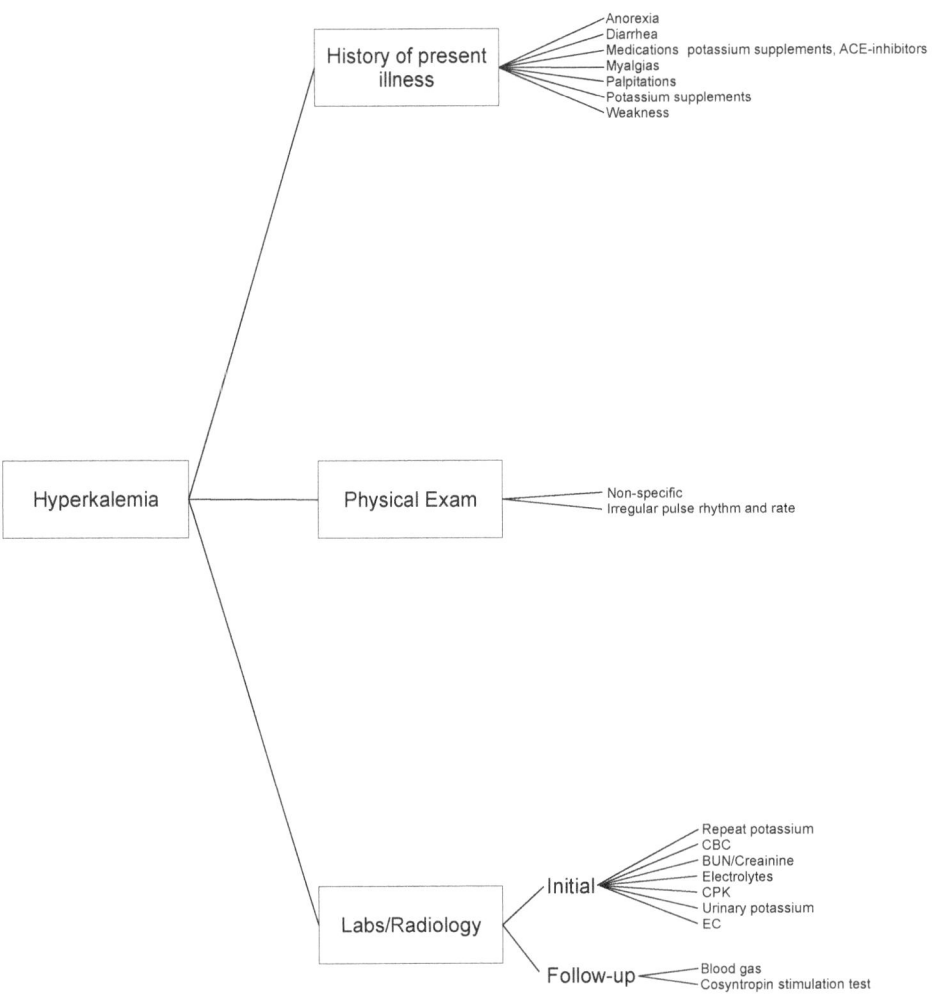

Hyperkalemia

History of present illness
- Anorexia
- Diarrhea
- Medications  potassium supplements, ACE-inhibitors
- Myalgias
- Palpitations
- Potassium supplements
- Weakness

Physical Exam
- Non-specific
- Irregular pulse rhythm and rate

Labs/Radiology

Initial
- Repeat potassium
- CBC
- BUN/Creainine
- Electrolytes
- CPK
- Urinary potassium
- EC

Follow-up
- Blood gas
- Cosyntropin stimulation test

# Secondary Hypertension

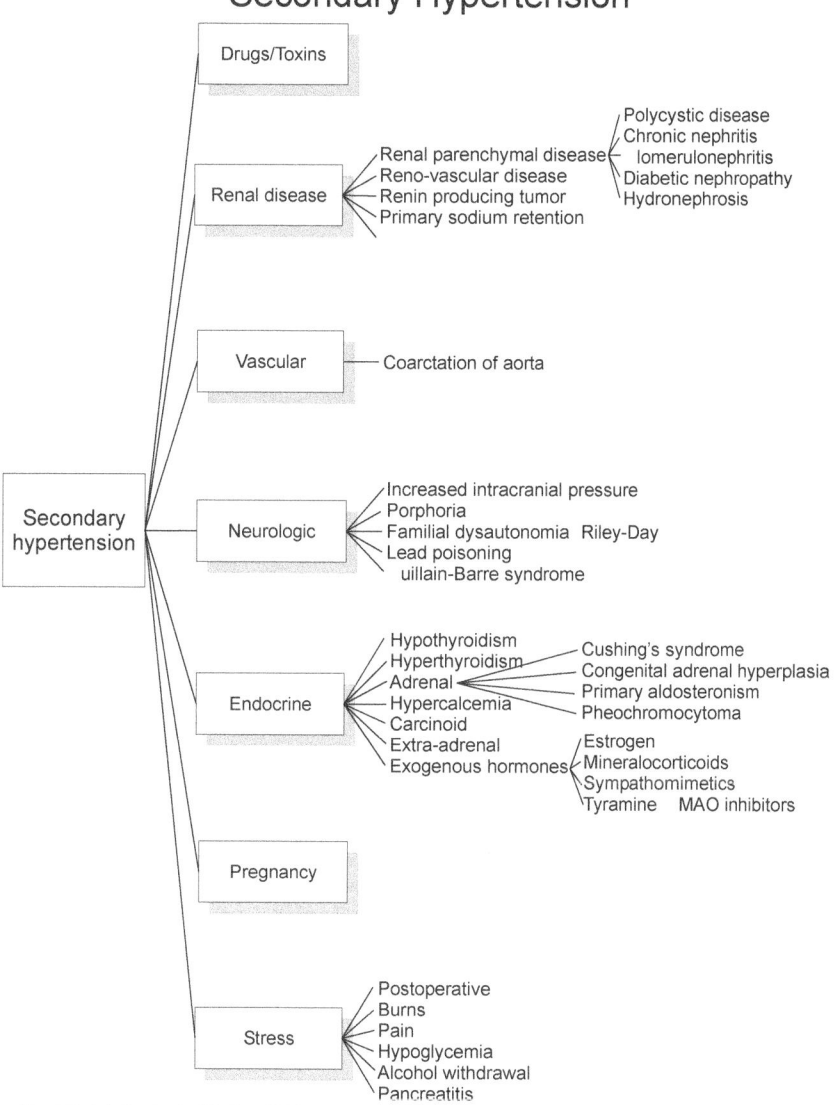

Drugs/Toxins

Renal disease
- Renal parenchymal disease
  - Polycystic disease
  - Chronic nephritis
  - Iomerulonephritis
  - Diabetic nephropathy
  - Hydronephrosis
- Reno-vascular disease
- Renin producing tumor
- Primary sodium retention

Vascular
- Coarctation of aorta

Neurologic
- Increased intracranial pressure
- Porphoria
- Familial dysautonomia  Riley-Day
- Lead poisoning
- uillain-Barre syndrome

Endocrine
- Hypothyroidism
- Hyperthyroidism
- Adrenal
  - Cushing's syndrome
  - Congenital adrenal hyperplasia
  - Primary aldosteronism
  - Pheochromocytoma
- Hypercalcemia
- Carcinoid
- Extra-adrenal
- Exogenous hormones
  - Estrogen
  - Mineralocorticoids
  - Sympathomimetics
  - Tyramine    MAO inhibitors

Pregnancy

Stress
- Postoperative
- Burns
- Pain
- Hypoglycemia
- Alcohol withdrawal
- Pancreatitis

Zoorob RJ, et al.  Hypertension. Prim Care. 2000 Sep;27(3):589-614,v.

# Hyperthyroidism

Hyperthyroidism

- raves' disease
- Toxic multinodular goiter
- Hyperfunctioning thyroid adenoma
- Exogenous hyperthyroidism
- Thyroiditis
- Other
  - Chorionic tumors
  - Struma ovarii
  - Thyroid carcinoma
  - Excess TSH secretion

Reference: Lazarus J. Hyperthyroidism. Lancet 1997;349:339-

# Hyperthyroidism

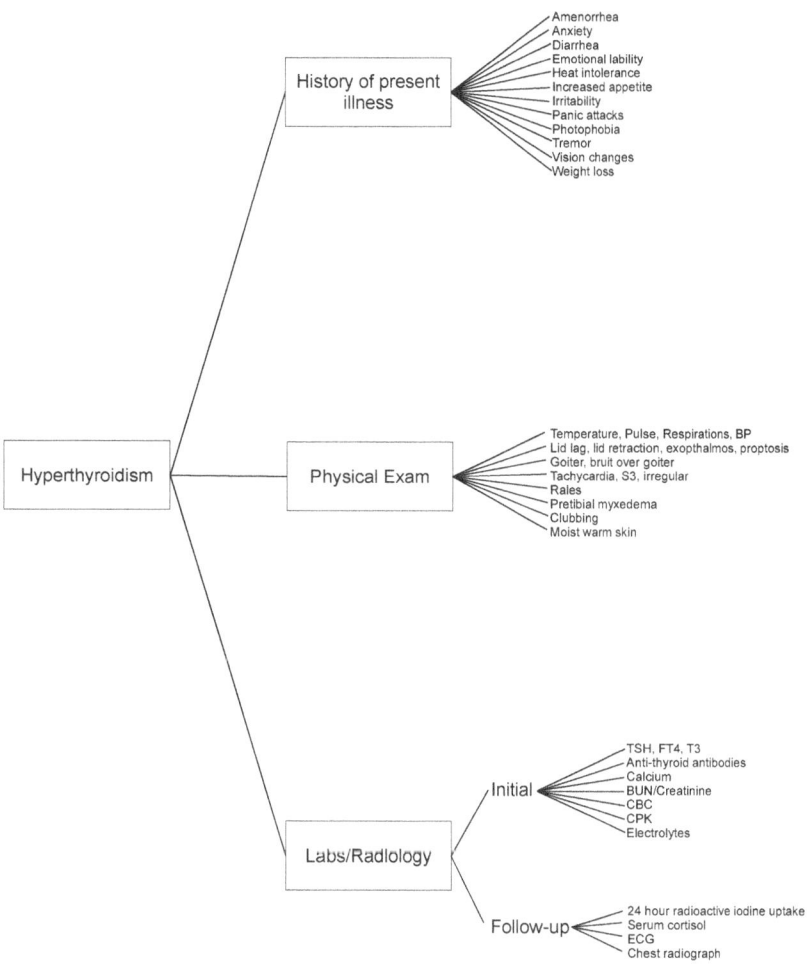

# Hypoalbuminemia

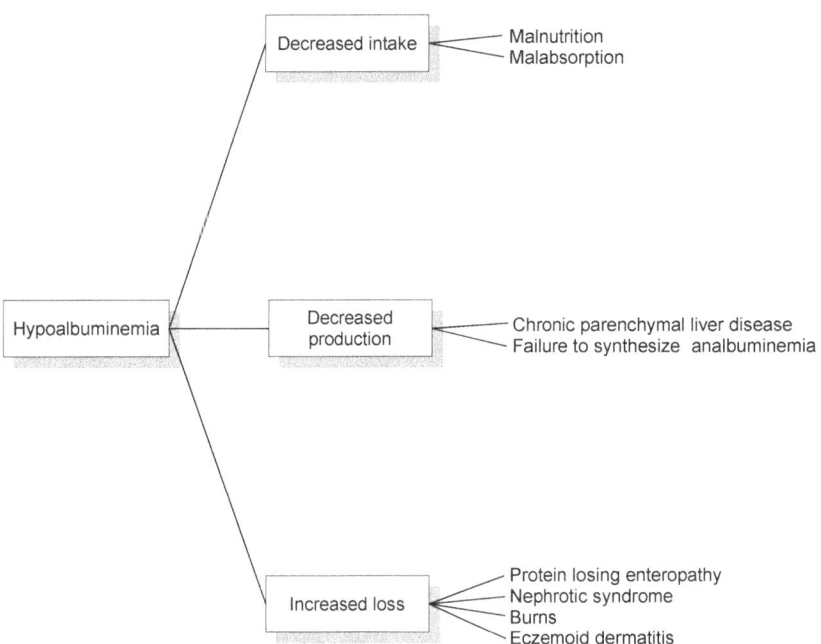

Hypoalbuminemia

Decreased intake
— Malnutrition
— Malabsorption

Decreased production
— Chronic parenchymal liver disease
— Failure to synthesize  analbuminemia

Increased loss
— Protein losing enteropathy
— Nephrotic syndrome
— Burns
— Eczemoid dermatitis

Reference: Emerson T. Unique features of albumin: a brief review. Crit Care Med 1989;17(7):690-4.

# Hypoalbuminemia

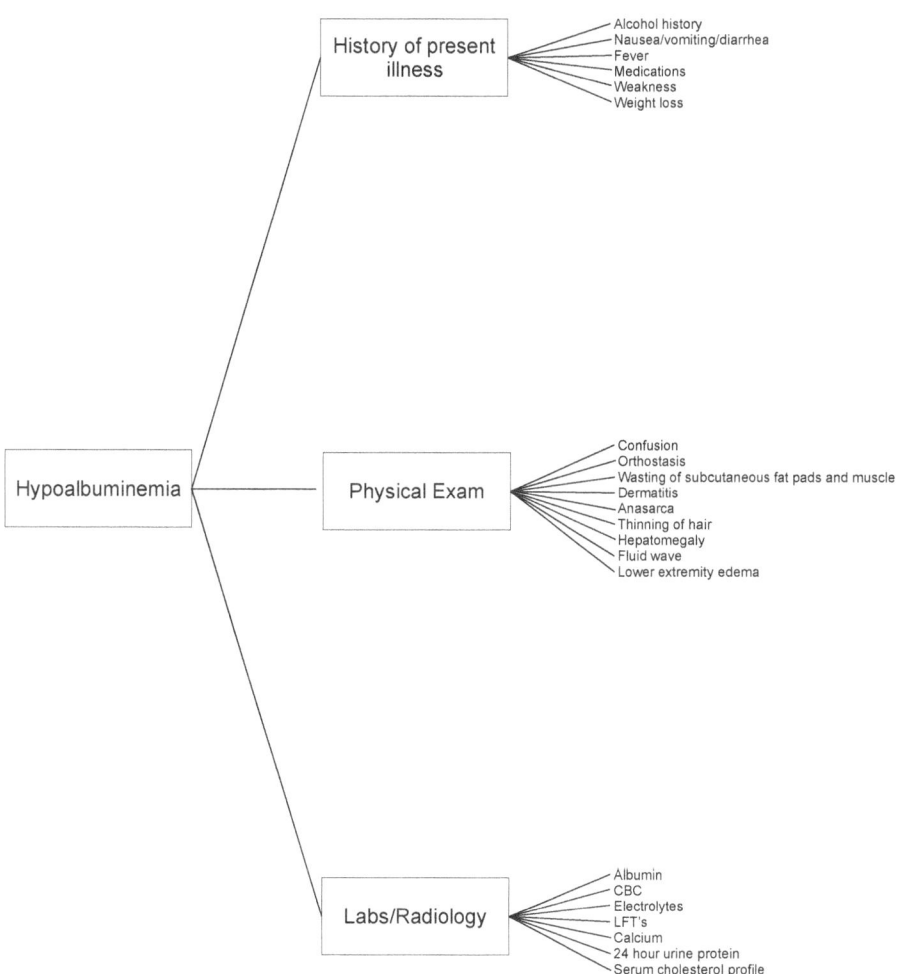

# Hypocalcemia

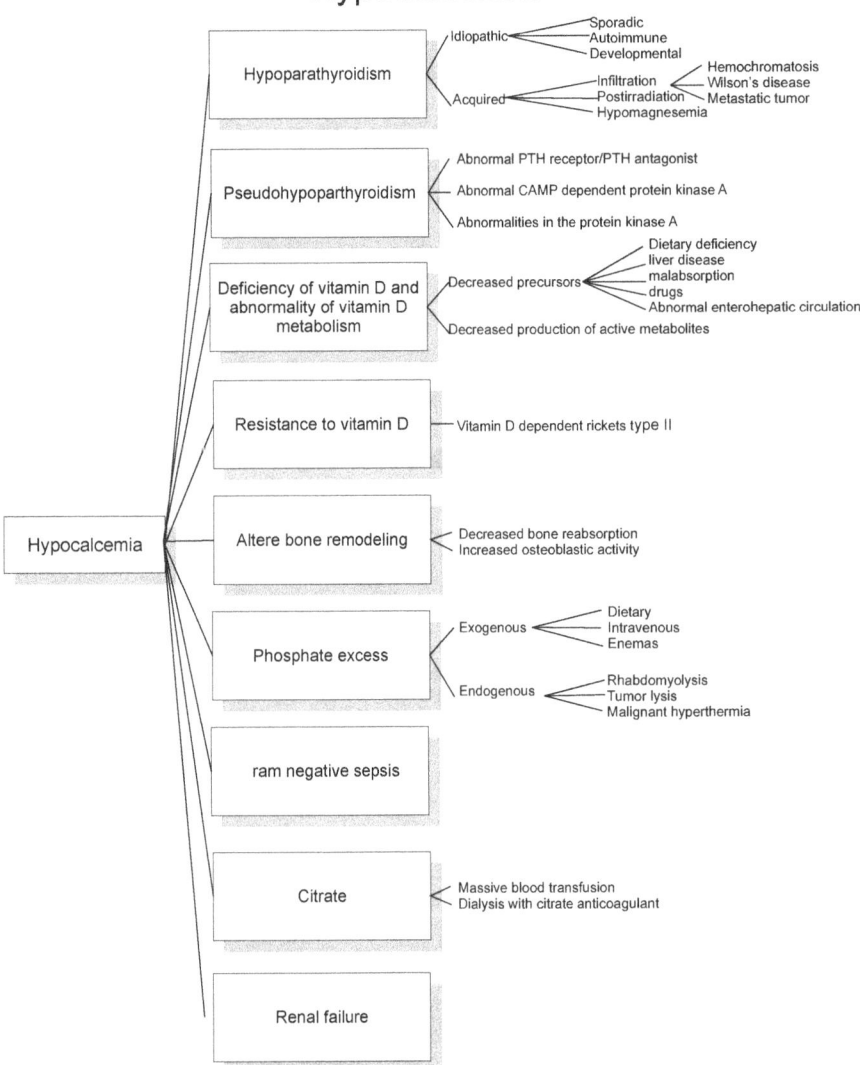

- **Hypoparathyroidism**
  - Idiopathic
    - Sporadic
    - Autoimmune
    - Developmental
  - Acquired
    - Infiltration
      - Hemochromatosis
      - Wilson's disease
      - Metastatic tumor
    - Postirradiation
    - Hypomagnesemia

- **Pseudohypoparthyroidism**
  - Abnormal PTH receptor/PTH antagonist
  - Abnormal CAMP dependent protein kinase A
  - Abnormalities in the protein kinase A

- **Deficiency of vitamin D and abnormality of vitamin D metabolism**
  - Decreased precursors
    - Dietary deficiency
    - liver disease
    - malabsorption
    - drugs
    - Abnormal enterohepatic circulation
  - Decreased production of active metabolites

- **Resistance to vitamin D**
  - Vitamin D dependent rickets type II

- **Altere bone remodeling**
  - Decreased bone reabsorption
  - Increased osteoblastic activity

- **Phosphate excess**
  - Exogenous
    - Dietary
    - Intravenous
    - Enemas
  - Endogenous
    - Rhabdomyolysis
    - Tumor lysis
    - Malignant hyperthermia

- **ram negative sepsis**

- **Citrate**
  - Massive blood transfusion
  - Dialysis with citrate anticoagulant

- **Renal failure**

Reference: Bushinsky D, Monk R. Calcium. Lancet 1998;352(9124):306-11.R

# Hypocalcemia

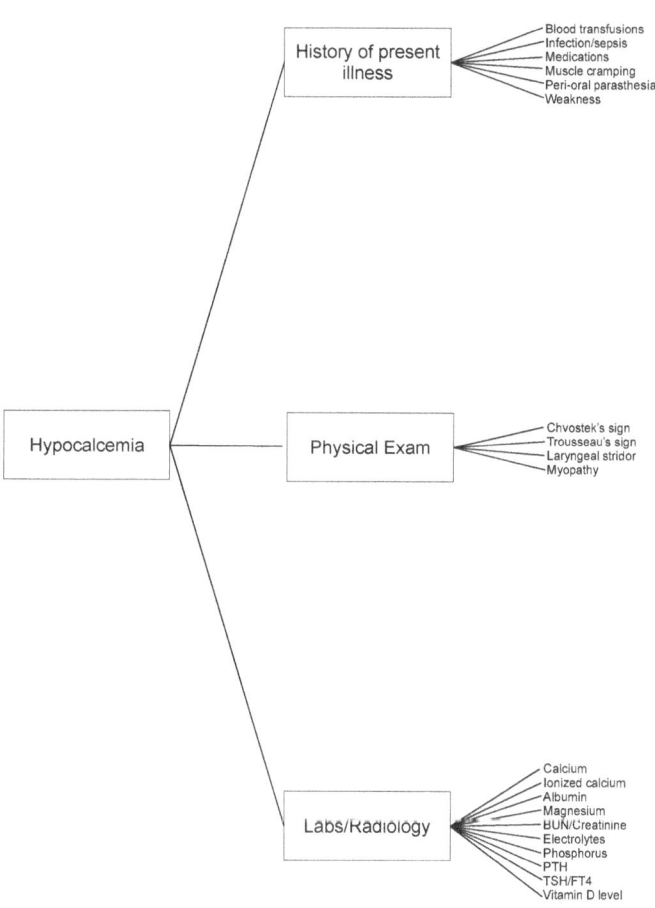

# Hypomagnesemia

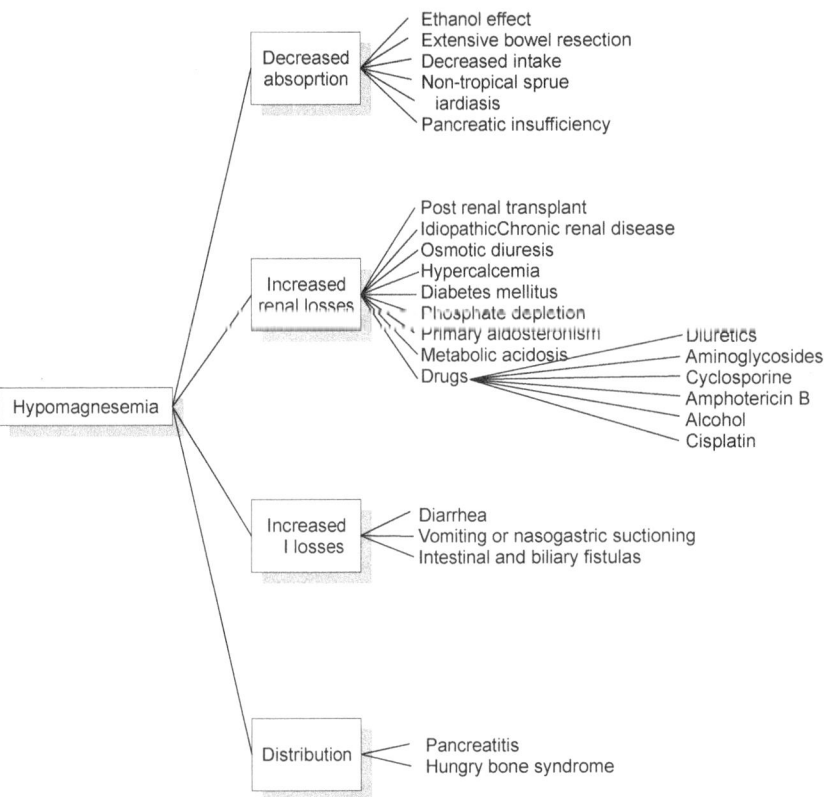

Reference: Swain R, Kaplan-Machlis B. Magnesium for the next millenium. South Med J 1999;92(11):1040-7.

# Hypomagnesemia

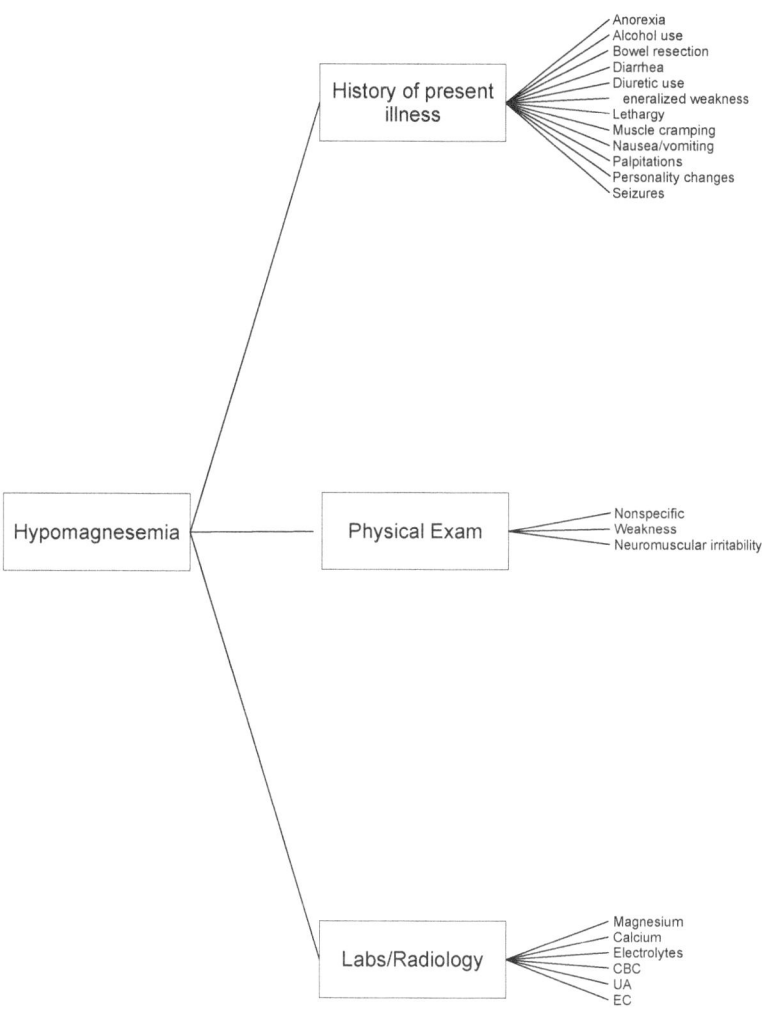

**Hypomagnesemia**

**History of present illness**
- Anorexia
- Alcohol use
- Bowel resection
- Diarrhea
- Diuretic use
- eneralized weakness
- Lethargy
- Muscle cramping
- Nausea/vomiting
- Palpitations
- Personality changes
- Seizures

**Physical Exam**
- Nonspecific
- Weakness
- Neuromuscular irritability

**Labs/Radiology**
- Magnesium
- Calcium
- Electrolytes
- CBC
- UA
- EC

# HYPONATREMIA

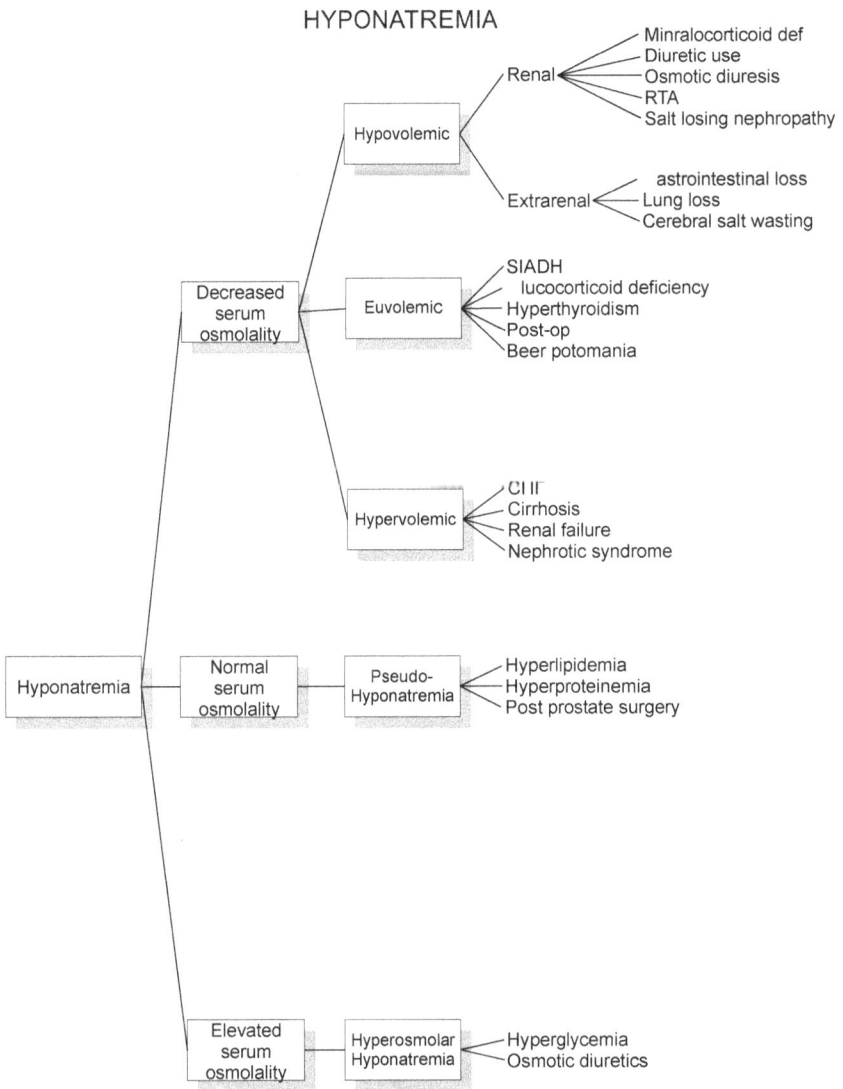

Reference: Miller M. Hyponatremia: Age-related risk factors and therapy decisions. Geriatrics 1998;53(7):32-3,37-8,41-2.

# Hyponatremia

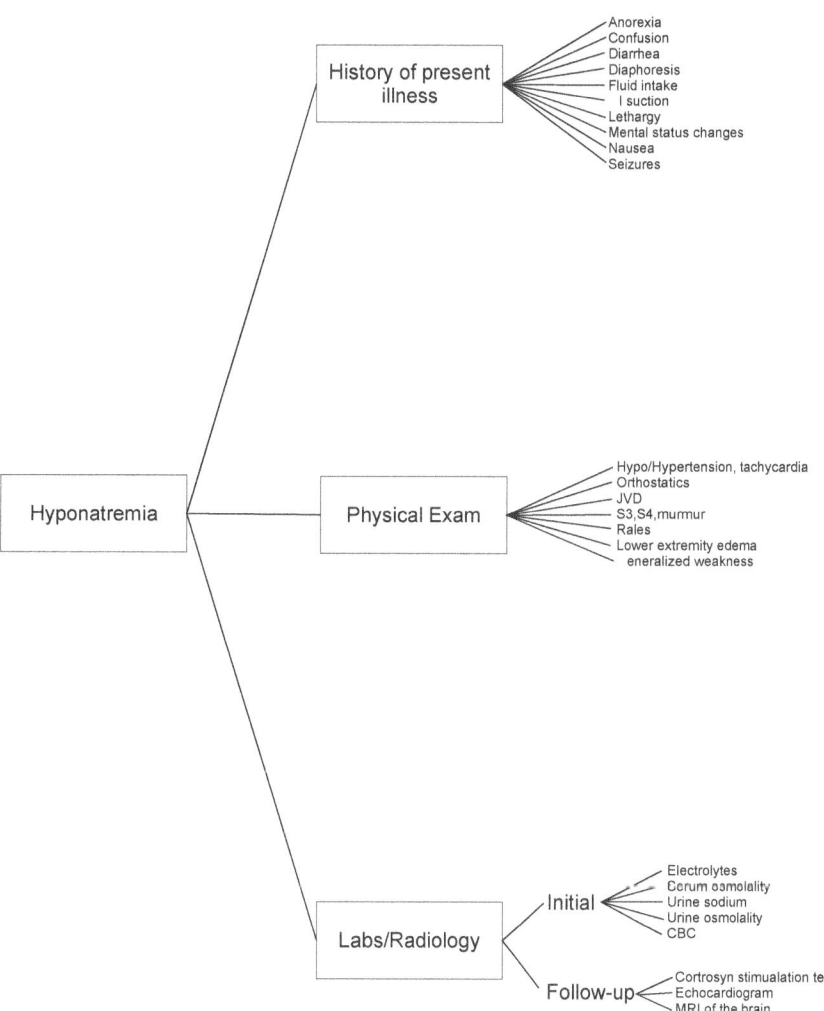

**Hyponatremia**

**History of present illness**
- Anorexia
- Confusion
- Diarrhea
- Diaphoresis
- Fluid intake
- I suction
- Lethargy
- Mental status changes
- Nausea
- Seizures

**Physical Exam**
- Hypo/Hypertension, tachycardia
- Orthostatics
- JVD
- S3,S4,murmur
- Rales
- Lower extremity edema
- eneralized weakness

**Labs/Radiology**

Initial
- Electrolytes
- Serum osmolality
- Urine sodium
- Urine osmolality
- CBC

Follow-up
- Cortrosyn stimualation test
- Echocardiogram
- MRI of the brain

# Hypothyroidism

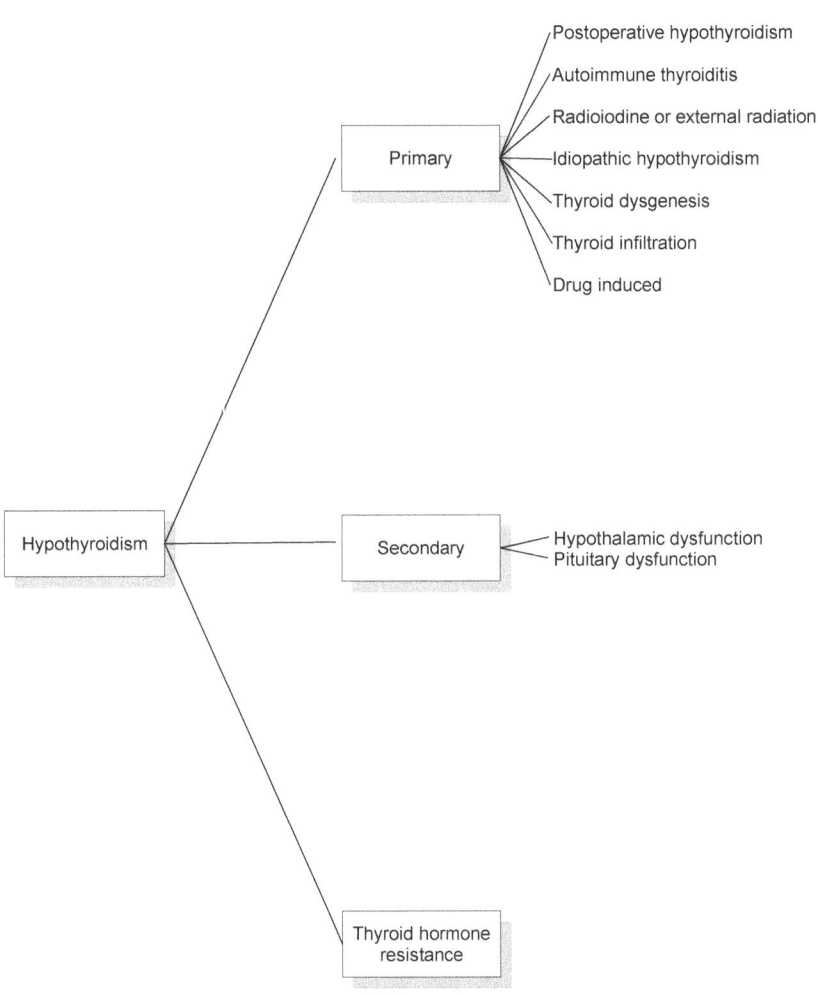

Primary
- Postoperative hypothyroidism
- Autoimmune thyroiditis
- Radioiodine or external radiation
- Idiopathic hypothyroidism
- Thyroid dysgenesis
- Thyroid infiltration
- Drug induced

Secondary
- Hypothalamic dysfunction
- Pituitary dysfunction

Thyroid hormone resistance

Lazarus JH, et al. Thyroid disorders --an update.Postgrad Med J. 2000 Sep;76(899):529-36.

# Hypothyroidism

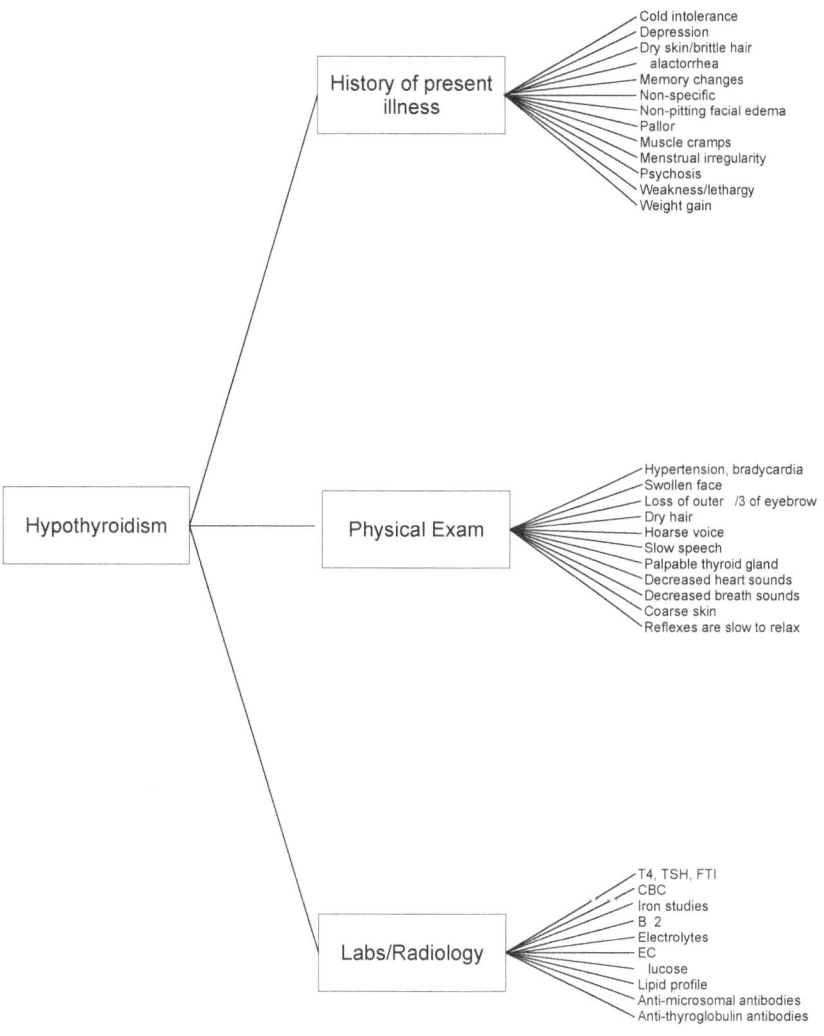

**Hypothyroidism**

**History of present illness**
- Cold intolerance
- Depression
- Dry skin/brittle hair
- alactorrhea
- Memory changes
- Non-specific
- Non-pitting facial edema
- Pallor
- Muscle cramps
- Menstrual irregularity
- Psychosis
- Weakness/lethargy
- Weight gain

**Physical Exam**
- Hypertension, bradycardia
- Swollen face
- Loss of outer /3 of eyebrow
- Dry hair
- Hoarse voice
- Slow speech
- Palpable thyroid gland
- Decreased heart sounds
- Decreased breath sounds
- Coarse skin
- Reflexes are slow to relax

**Labs/Radiology**
- T4, TSH, FTI
- CBC
- Iron studies
- B 2
- Electrolytes
- EC
- lucose
- Lipid profile
- Anti-microsomal antibodies
- Anti-thyroglobulin antibodies

# Jaundice

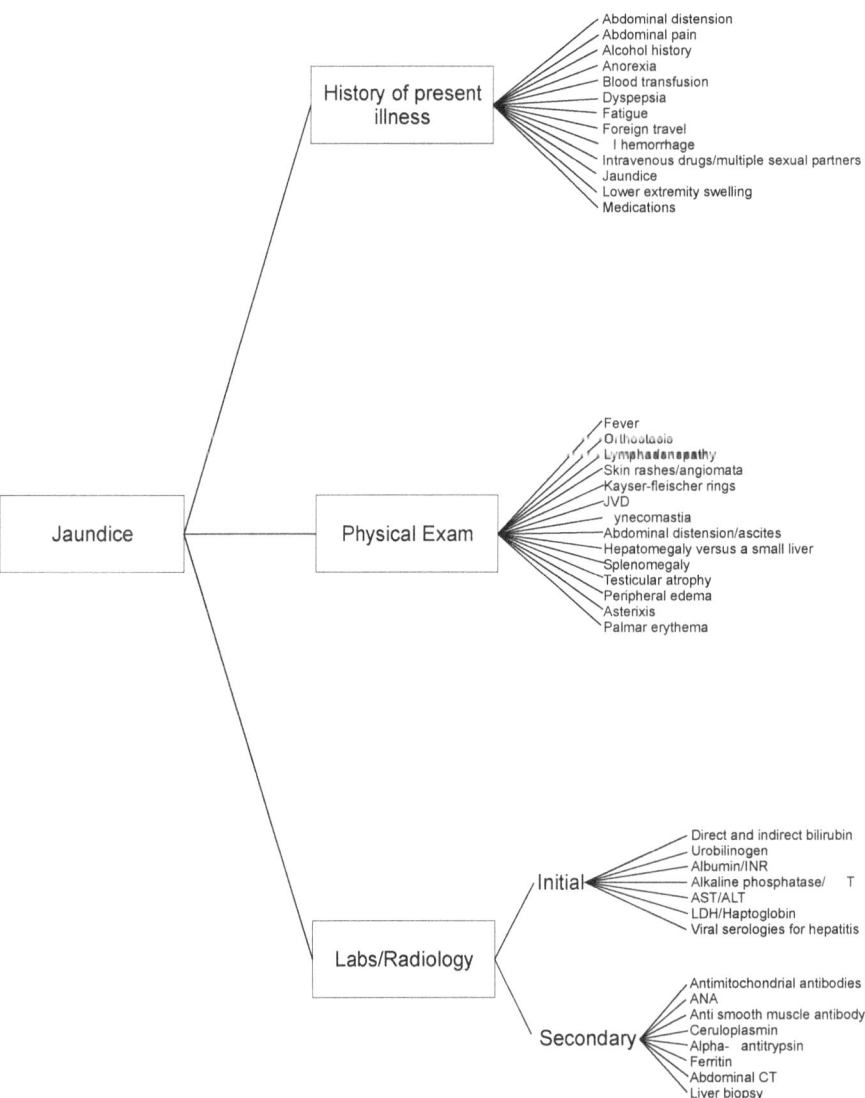

Jaundice

History of present illness
- Abdominal distension
- Abdominal pain
- Alcohol history
- Anorexia
- Blood transfusion
- Dyspepsia
- Fatigue
- Foreign travel
- I hemorrhage
- Intravenous drugs/multiple sexual partners
- Jaundice
- Lower extremity swelling
- Medications

Physical Exam
- Fever
- Orthostasis
- Lymphadenopathy
- Skin rashes/angiomata
- Kayser-fleischer rings
- JVD
- ynecomastia
- Abdominal distension/ascites
- Hepatomegaly versus a small liver
- Splenomegaly
- Testicular atrophy
- Peripheral edema
- Asterixis
- Palmar erythema

Labs/Radiology

Initial
- Direct and indirect bilirubin
- Urobilinogen
- Albumin/INR
- Alkaline phosphatase/    T
- AST/ALT
- LDH/Haptoglobin
- Viral serologies for hepatitis

Secondary
- Antimitochondrial antibodies
- ANA
- Anti smooth muscle antibody
- Ceruloplasmin
- Alpha-  antitrypsin
- Ferritin
- Abdominal CT
- Liver biopsy

# Lactic Acidosis

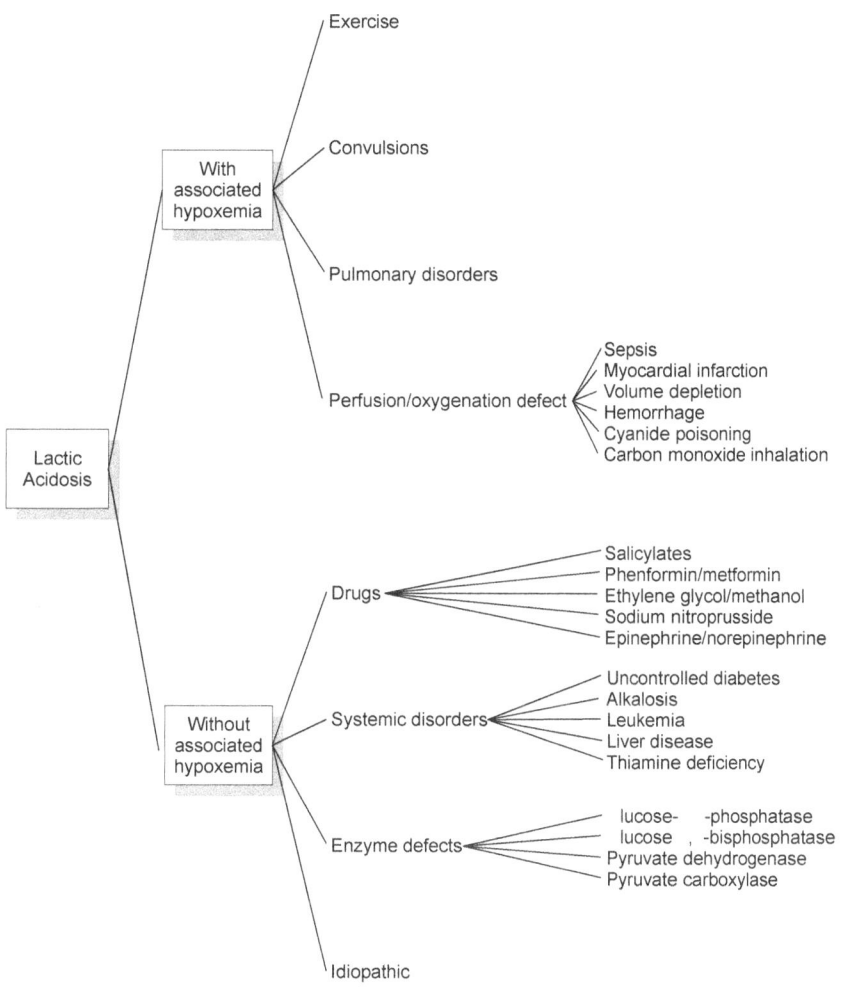

- With associated hypoxemia
  - Exercise
  - Convulsions
  - Pulmonary disorders
  - Perfusion/oxygenation defect
    - Sepsis
    - Myocardial infarction
    - Volume depletion
    - Hemorrhage
    - Cyanide poisoning
    - Carbon monoxide inhalation

- Lactic Acidosis

- Without associated hypoxemia
  - Drugs
    - Salicylates
    - Phenformin/metformin
    - Ethylene glycol/methanol
    - Sodium nitroprusside
    - Epinephrine/norepinephrine
  - Systemic disorders
    - Uncontrolled diabetes
    - Alkalosis
    - Leukemia
    - Liver disease
    - Thiamine deficiency
  - Enzyme defects
    - lucose-    -phosphatase
    - lucose   , -bisphosphatase
    - Pyruvate dehydrogenase
    - Pyruvate carboxylase
  - Idiopathic

Reference: Kelley, Essentials In Internal Medicine, ed 3, Philadelphia, 1994,J B. Lippincott, page 262

Isselbacher K, Braunwald E, Wilson J, Martin J, Fauci Am Kasper D, Harrison's Principles of Internal Medicine, ed  3, New  ork,    4, Mcgraw Hill Book Company  Page 2

# Lactic Acidosis

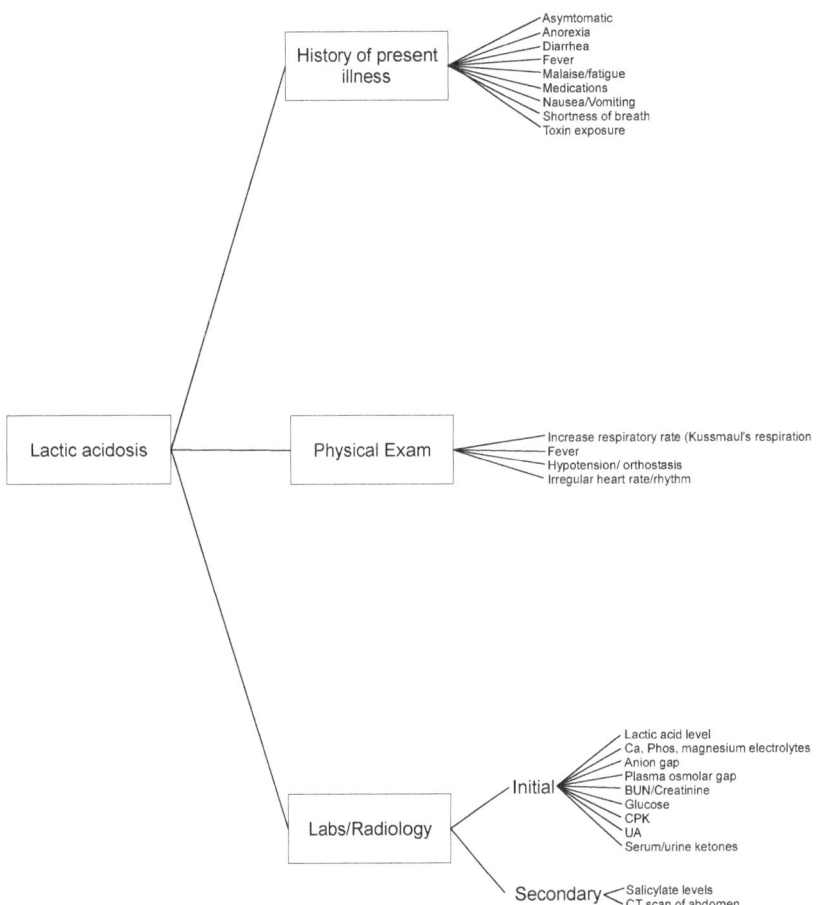

Lactic acidosis

History of present illness
- Asymtomatic
- Anorexia
- Diarrhea
- Fever
- Malaise/fatigue
- Medications
- Nausea/Vomiting
- Shortness of breath
- Toxin exposure

Physical Exam
- Increase respiratory rate (Kussmaul's respiration
- Fever
- Hypotension/ orthostasis
- Irregular heart rate/rhythm

Labs/Radiology

Initial
- Lactic acid level
- Ca, Phos, magnesium electrolytes
- Anion gap
- Plasma osmolar gap
- BUN/Creatinine
- Glucose
- CPK
- UA
- Serum/urine ketones

Secondary
- Salicylate levels
- CT scan of abdomen

# Change in Mental Status

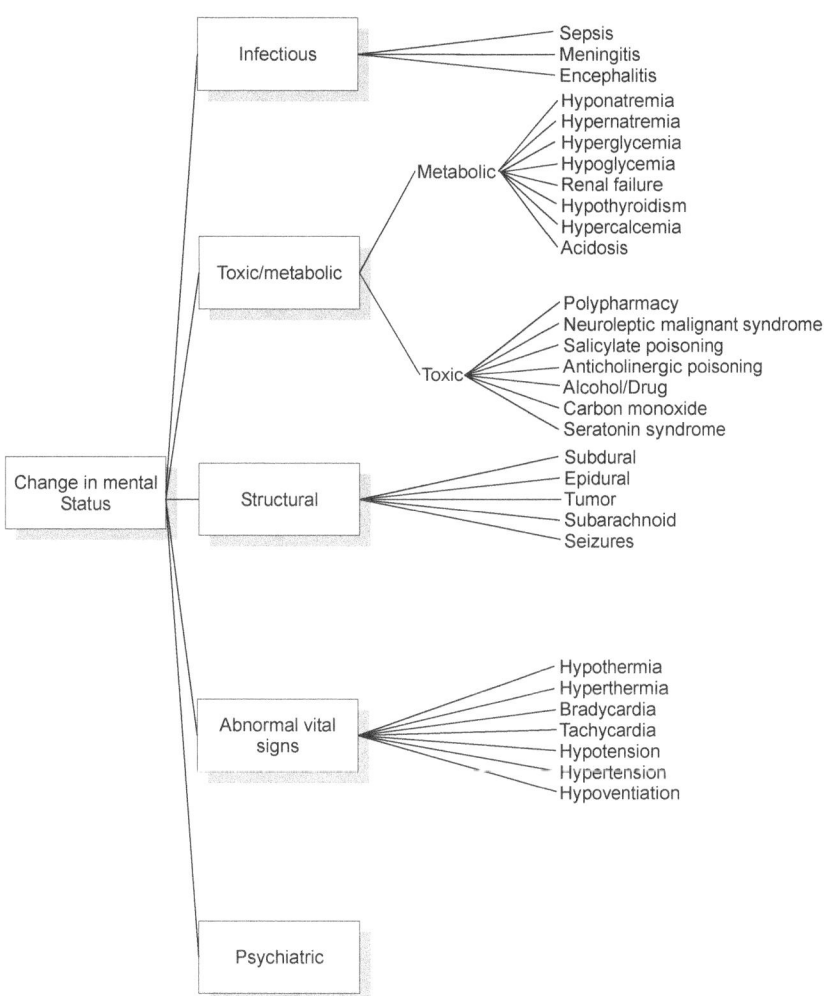

Reference: O'Keefe K, Sanson T: Elderly patients with change in mental status. Emergency Medicine Clinics of North America16(4):701-15,1998.

# Acute Mental Status Changes

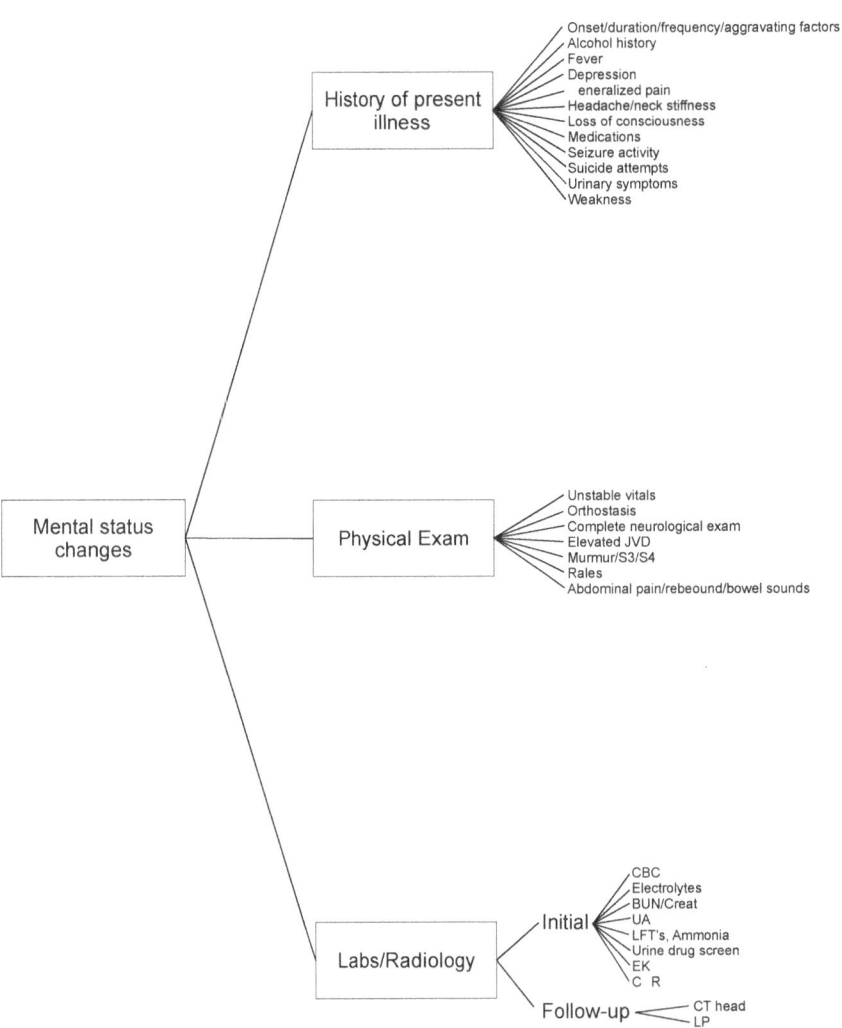

# Neutropenia

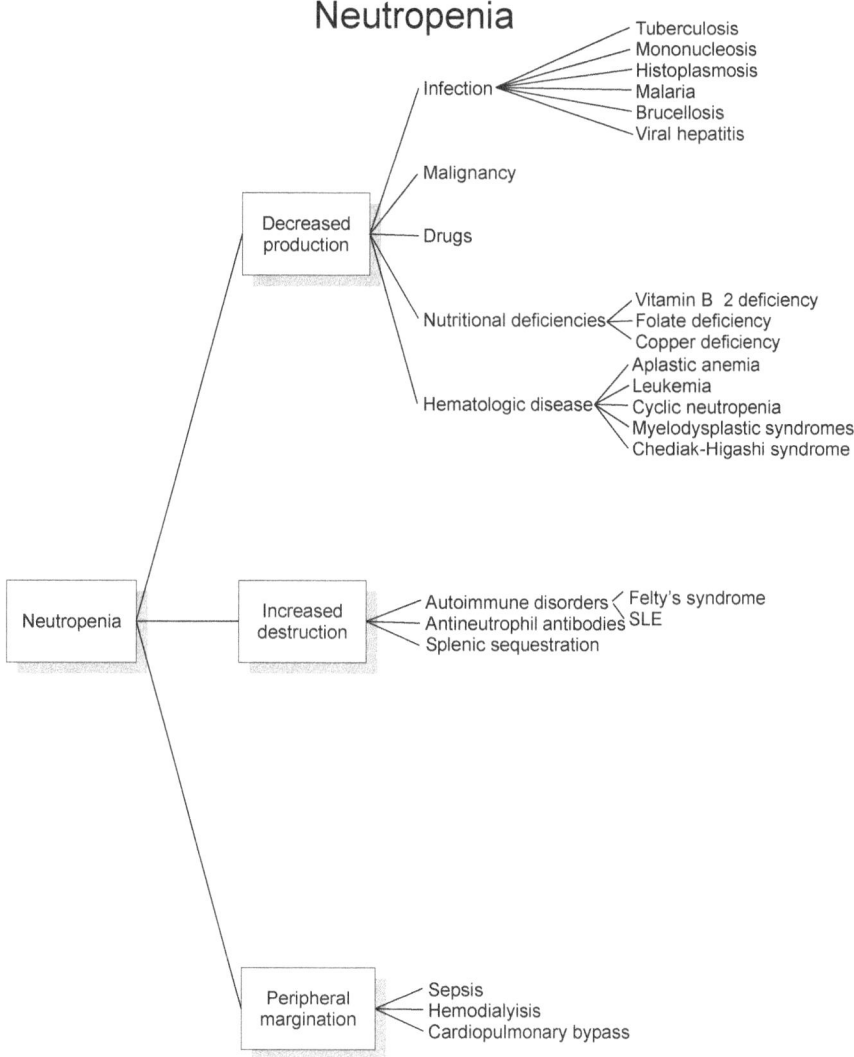

Infection
- Tuberculosis
- Mononucleosis
- Histoplasmosis
- Malaria
- Brucellosis
- Viral hepatitis

Decreased production
- Infection
- Malignancy
- Drugs
- Nutritional deficiencies
  - Vitamin B 2 deficiency
  - Folate deficiency
  - Copper deficiency
- Hematologic disease
  - Aplastic anemia
  - Leukemia
  - Cyclic neutropenia
  - Myelodysplastic syndromes
  - Chediak-Higashi syndrome

Neutropenia

Increased destruction
- Autoimmune disorders
  - Felty's syndrome
  - SLE
- Antineutrophil antibodies
- Splenic sequestration

Peripheral margination
- Sepsis
- Hemodialyisis
- Cardiopulmonary bypass

Reference: Russin S. Fillipo B. Adler A. Neutropenia in adults. What is its clinical significance? Postgrad Med 1990;88(2):209 16.

# Neutropenia

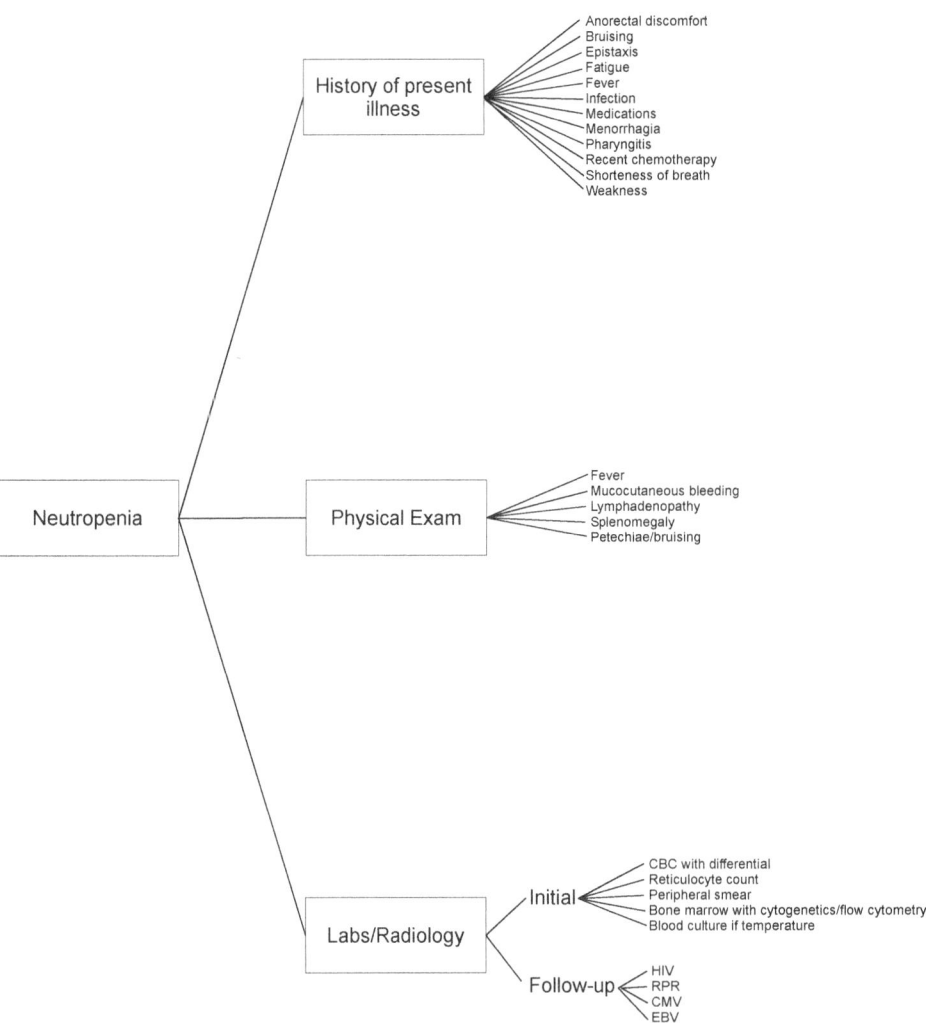

# Pacemaker Code

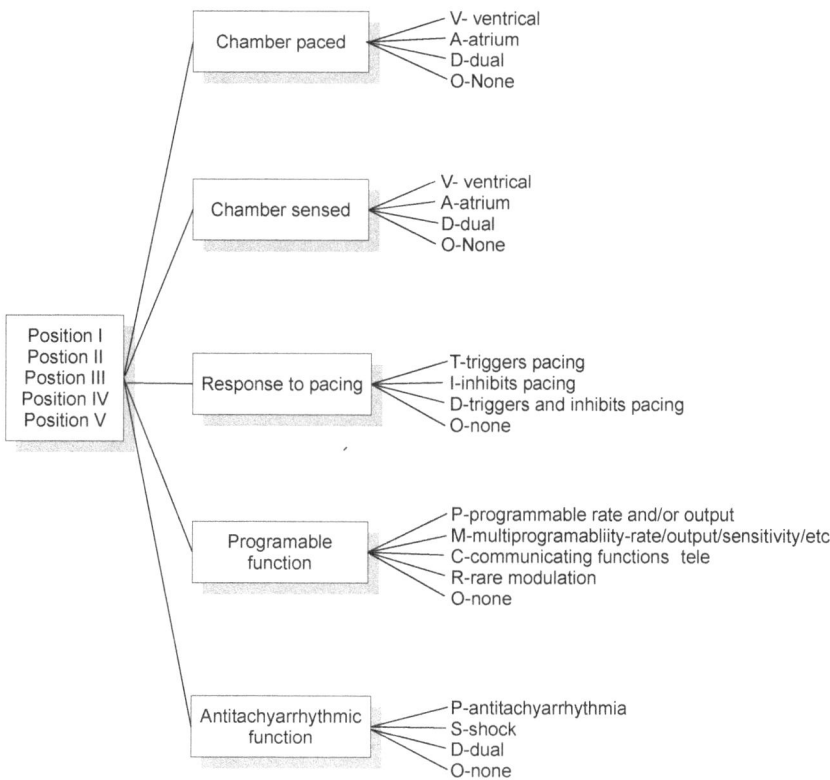

Reference: Barold S. Cardiac pacing in special and complex situations. Indications and modes of stimulation. Cardiol Clin 1992;10(4):573-91

# Acute Pancreatitis

Alcohol

Biliary stones

Medications
- Thiazide diuretics
- Sulfonamides
- Tetracycline
- Estrogens
- Azathiaprine
- Valproic acid
- Furosemide

Renal failure

Duodenal ulcer

Post-operative

ERCP

Metabolic disorders
- Hypertriglyceridemia
- Hypercalcemia

Pancrease divisum

Parasites

Scorpion bites

Collagen-vascular

Trauma

Ischemia/ hypotension

Hereditary
- Mumps
- Coxsackie virus
- Viral hepatitis
- Mycoplasma

Infectious

Reference  Kelley, Essentials In Internal Medicine, ed 3  Philadelphia,      4,J B  Lippincott, page  33

# Pancreatitis

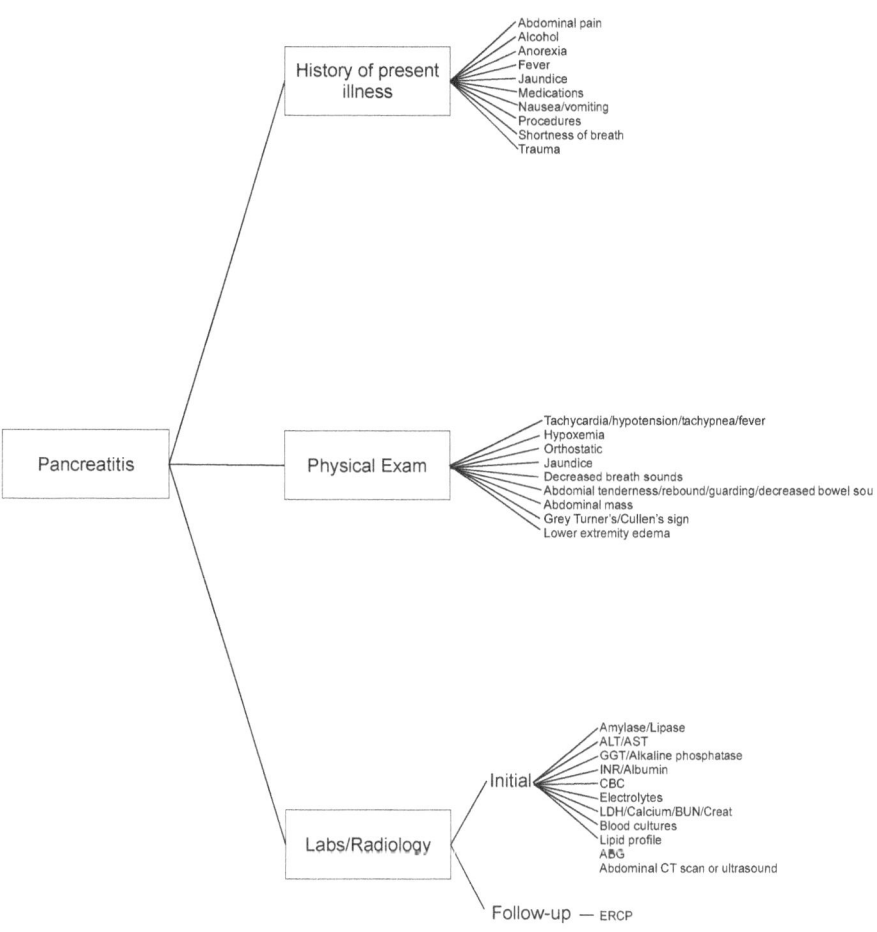

# Pulseless Electrical Activity

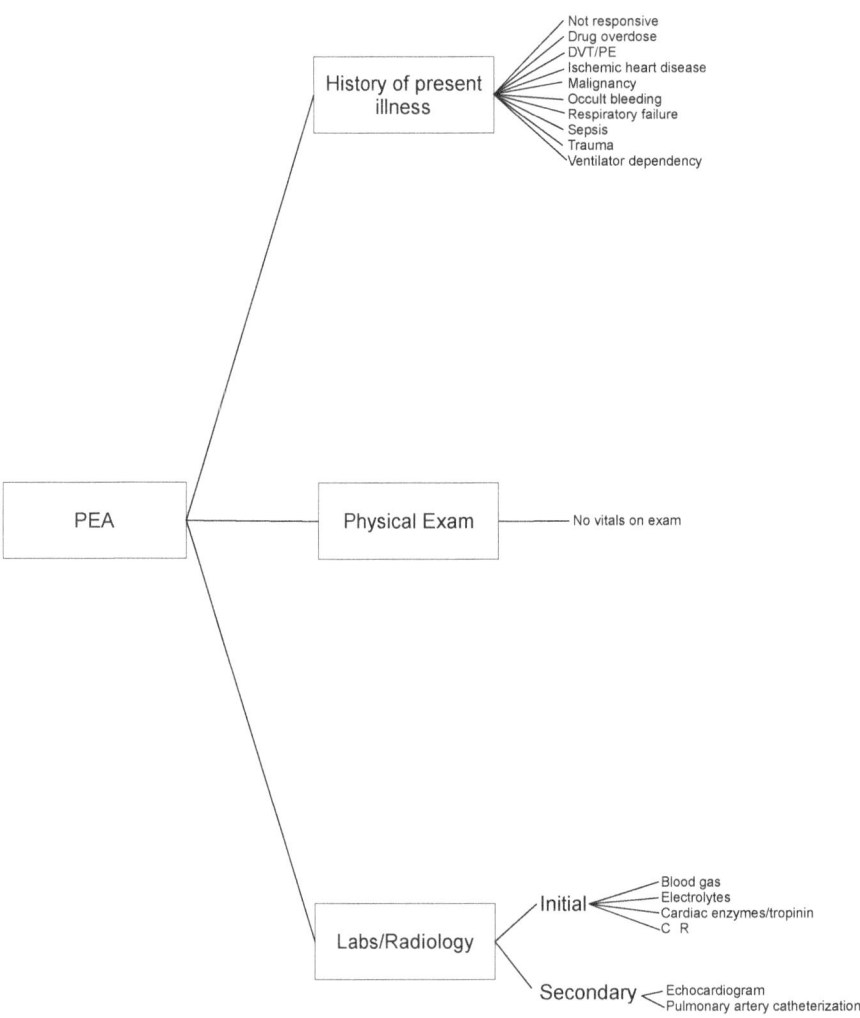

# Pericarditis

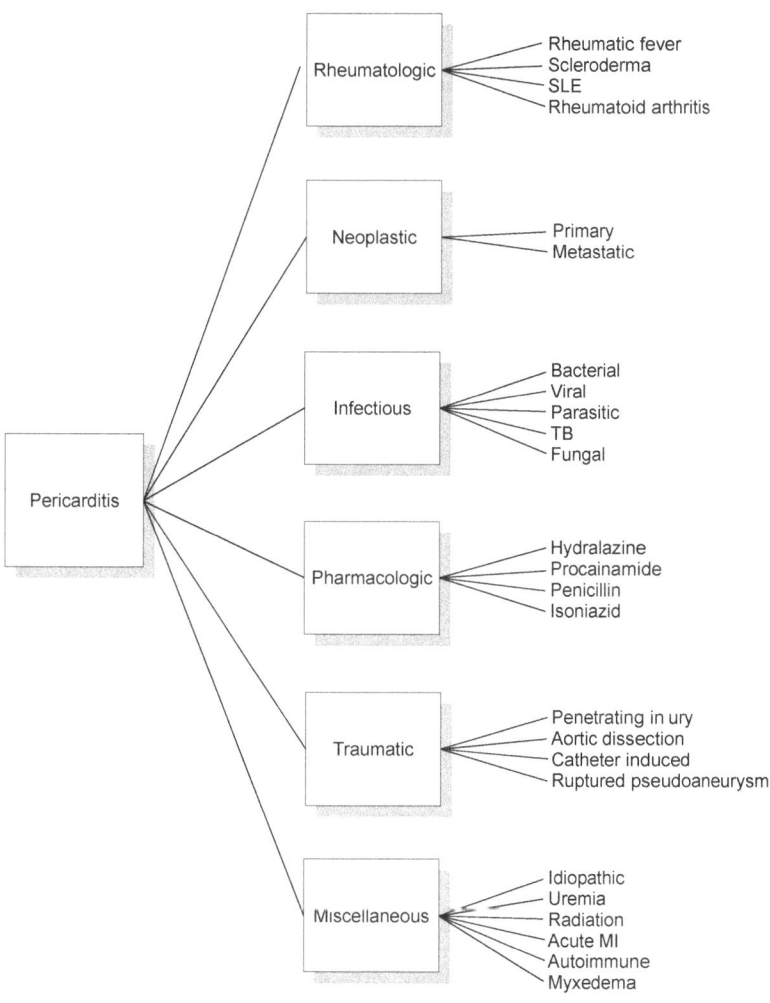

Reference: Marinella M. Electrocardiographic manifestations and differential diagnosis of acute pericarditis. American Family Physician 1998;57(4): 699-704

# Pericarditis

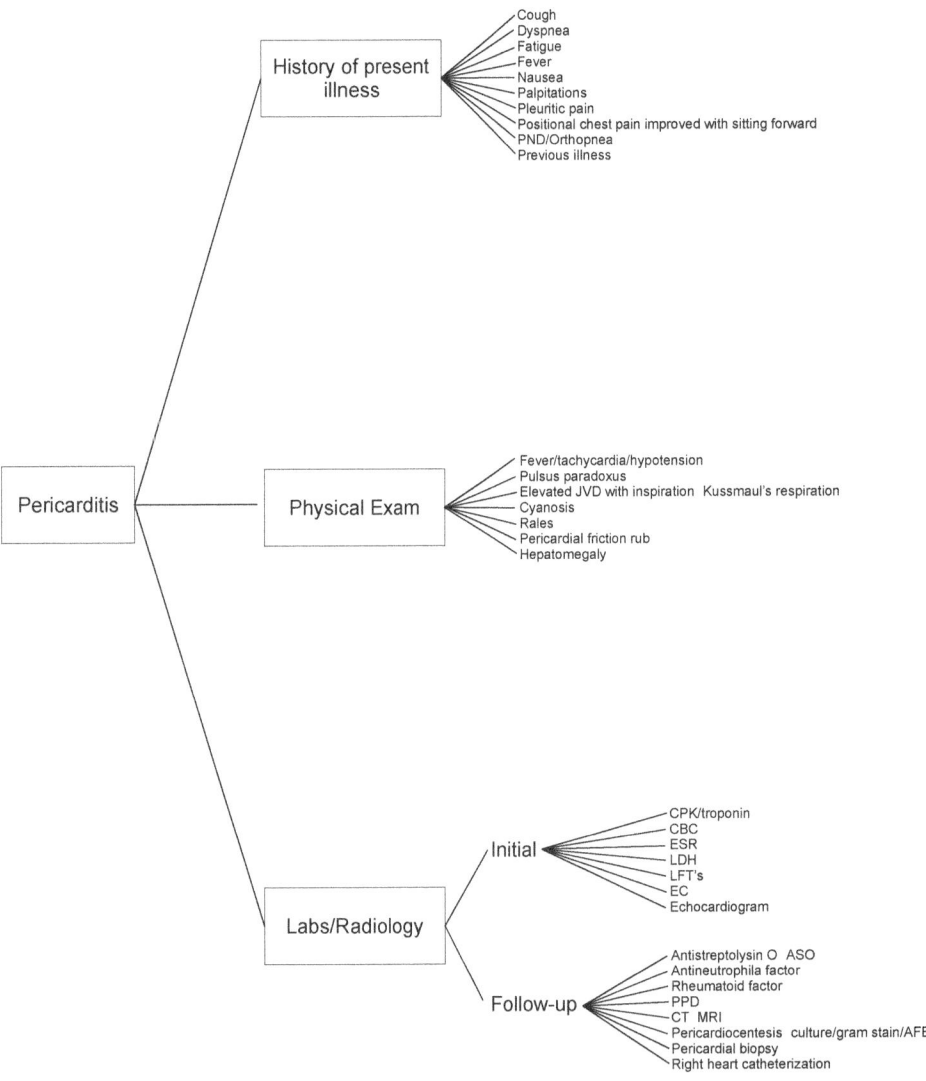

**Pericarditis**

**History of present illness**
- Cough
- Dyspnea
- Fatigue
- Fever
- Nausea
- Palpitations
- Pleuritic pain
- Positional chest pain improved with sitting forward
- PND/Orthopnea
- Previous illness

**Physical Exam**
- Fever/tachycardia/hypotension
- Pulsus paradoxus
- Elevated JVD with inspiration  Kussmaul's respiration
- Cyanosis
- Rales
- Pericardial friction rub
- Hepatomegaly

**Labs/Radiology**

Initial
- CPK/troponin
- CBC
- ESR
- LDH
- LFT's
- EC
- Echocardiogram

Follow-up
- Antistreptolysin O  ASO
- Antineutrophila factor
- Rheumatoid factor
- PPD
- CT  MRI
- Pericardiocentesis  culture/gram stain/AFB
- Pericardial biopsy
- Right heart catheterization

# Adrenal Insufficiency

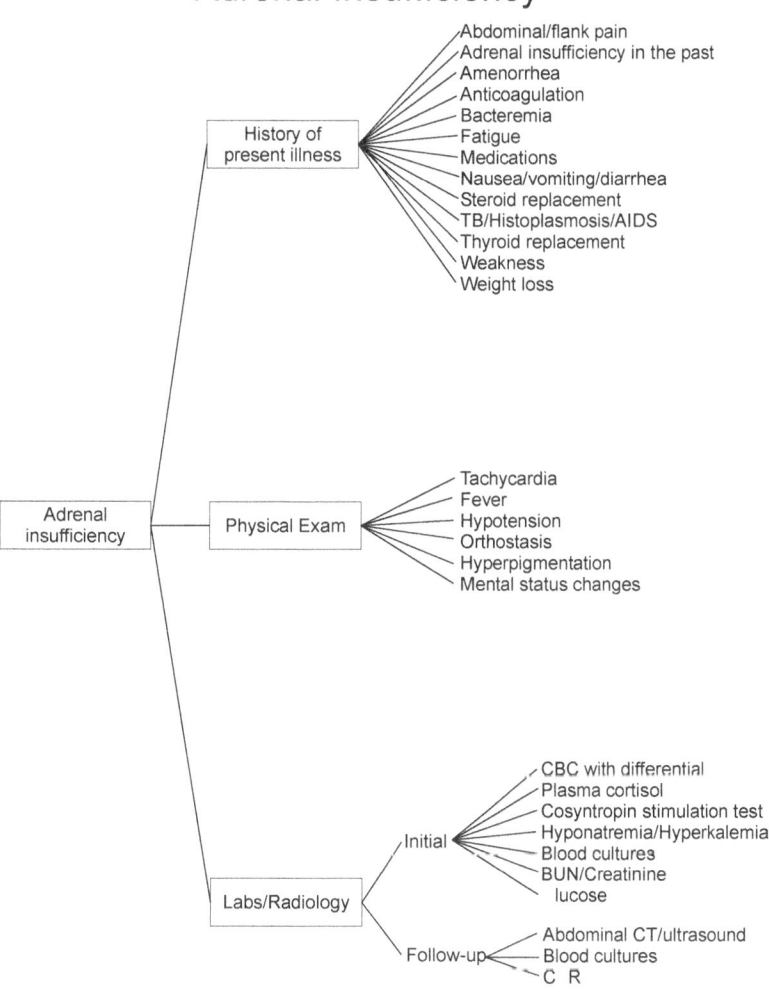

**Adrenal insufficiency**

**History of present illness**
- Abdominal/flank pain
- Adrenal insufficiency in the past
- Amenorrhea
- Anticoagulation
- Bacteremia
- Fatigue
- Medications
- Nausea/vomiting/diarrhea
- Steroid replacement
- TB/Histoplasmosis/AIDS
- Thyroid replacement
- Weakness
- Weight loss

**Physical Exam**
- Tachycardia
- Fever
- Hypotension
- Orthostasis
- Hyperpigmentation
- Mental status changes

**Labs/Radiology**

Initial
- CBC with differential
- Plasma cortisol
- Cosyntropin stimulation test
- Hyponatremia/Hyperkalemia
- Blood cultures
- BUN/Creatinine
- lucose

Follow-up
- Abdominal CT/ultrasound
- Blood cultures
- C R

# Pleural Effusion

**Pleural Effusion**

**Transudate**
-Total protein >3.0
-Protein/serum protein <0.5
-LDH/Serum LDH <0.6
-Fluid LDH < 200

- Congestive heart failure
- Nephrotic syndrome
- Cirrhosis
- Volume overload
- Myxedema
- Peritoneal dialysis
- Superior vena caval obstructio

**Exudate**
-Protein/serum protein >0.5
-LDH/serum LDH > 0.6
-Total protein > 3 g

- Infectious
  - Bacterial
  - Fungal
  - Tuberculosis
- Immunologic
  - Rheumatoid arthritis
  - Post cardiac in ury syndrome
  - Sarcoid
  - SLE
- Malignancy
- Drug induced
  - Dantrolene
  - Nitrofurantoin
  - Amiodarone
  - Methotrexate
- Miscellaneuous
  - Pancreatitis
  - Intra-abdominal infection
  - Pulmonary emboli/ infarction
  - Asbestos exposure
  - Chylous or pseudochylous effusion

Reference  Light R, macgregor M, Luchsinger P, et al  Pleural effusions the diagnostic separation of transudates and exudates  Ann Intern Med     2     4     - 3

# Pleural Effusion

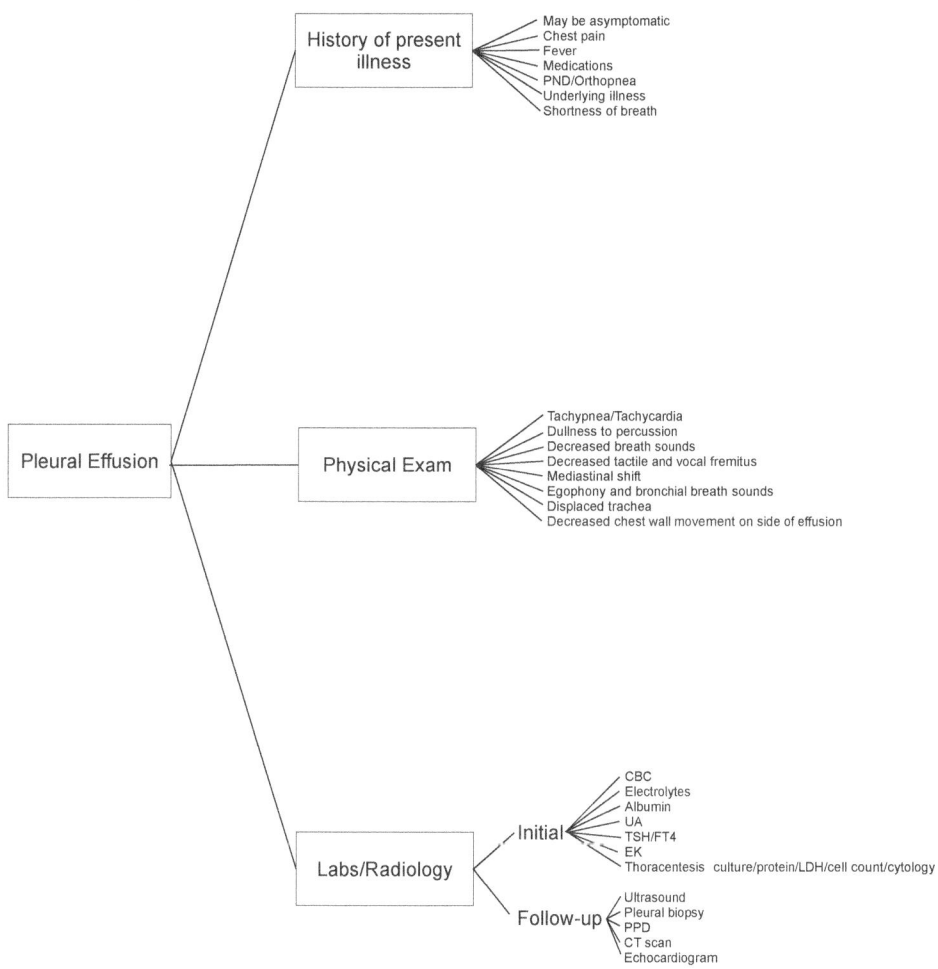

**Pleural Effusion**

**History of present illness**
- May be asymptomatic
- Chest pain
- Fever
- Medications
- PND/Orthopnea
- Underlying illness
- Shortness of breath

**Physical Exam**
- Tachypnea/Tachycardia
- Dullness to percussion
- Decreased breath sounds
- Decreased tactile and vocal fremitus
- Mediastinal shift
- Egophony and bronchial breath sounds
- Displaced trachea
- Decreased chest wall movement on side of effusion

**Labs/Radiology**

Initial
- CBC
- Electrolytes
- Albumin
- UA
- TSH/FT4
- EK
- Thoracentesis   culture/protein/LDH/cell count/cytology

Follow-up
- Ultrasound
- Pleural biopsy
- PPD
- CT scan
- Echocardiogram

# Pneumothorax

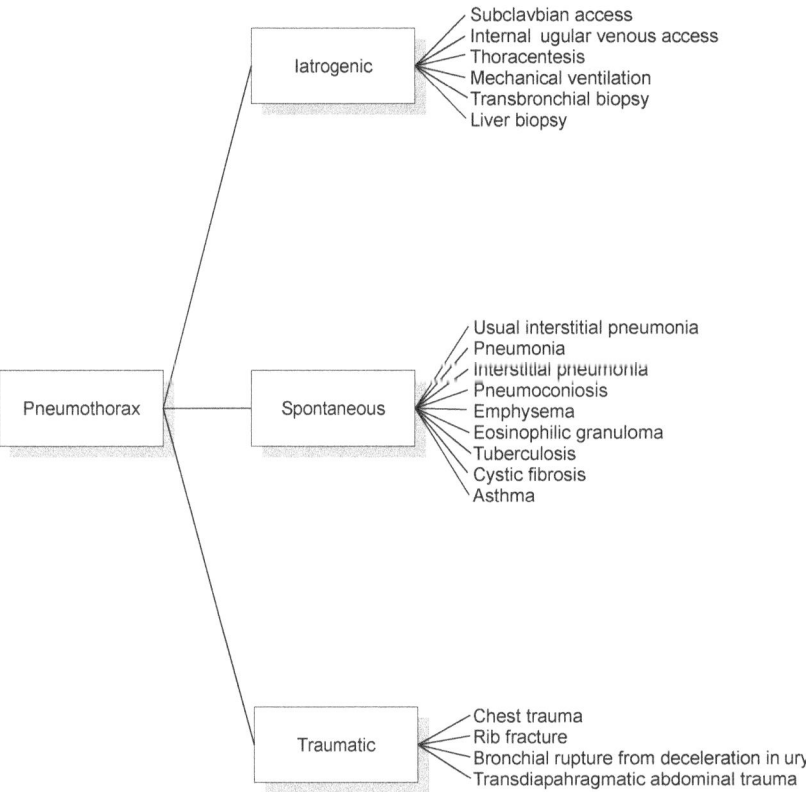

Pneumothorax

**Iatrogenic**
- Subclavbian access
- Internal ugular venous access
- Thoracentesis
- Mechanical ventilation
- Transbronchial biopsy
- Liver biopsy

**Spontaneous**
- Usual interstitial pneumonia
- Pneumonia
- Interstitial pneumonia
- Pneumoconiosis
- Emphysema
- Eosinophilic granuloma
- Tuberculosis
- Cystic fibrosis
- Asthma

**Traumatic**
- Chest trauma
- Rib fracture
- Bronchial rupture from deceleration in ury
- Transdiapahragmatic abdominal trauma

Reference: Andreili T, Bennett J, Carpenter C, Plum F, Smith L, Cecil Essentials of Medicine, ed 3, Philadelphia, 1993, W.B. Saunders Company. page 174

# Pneumothorax

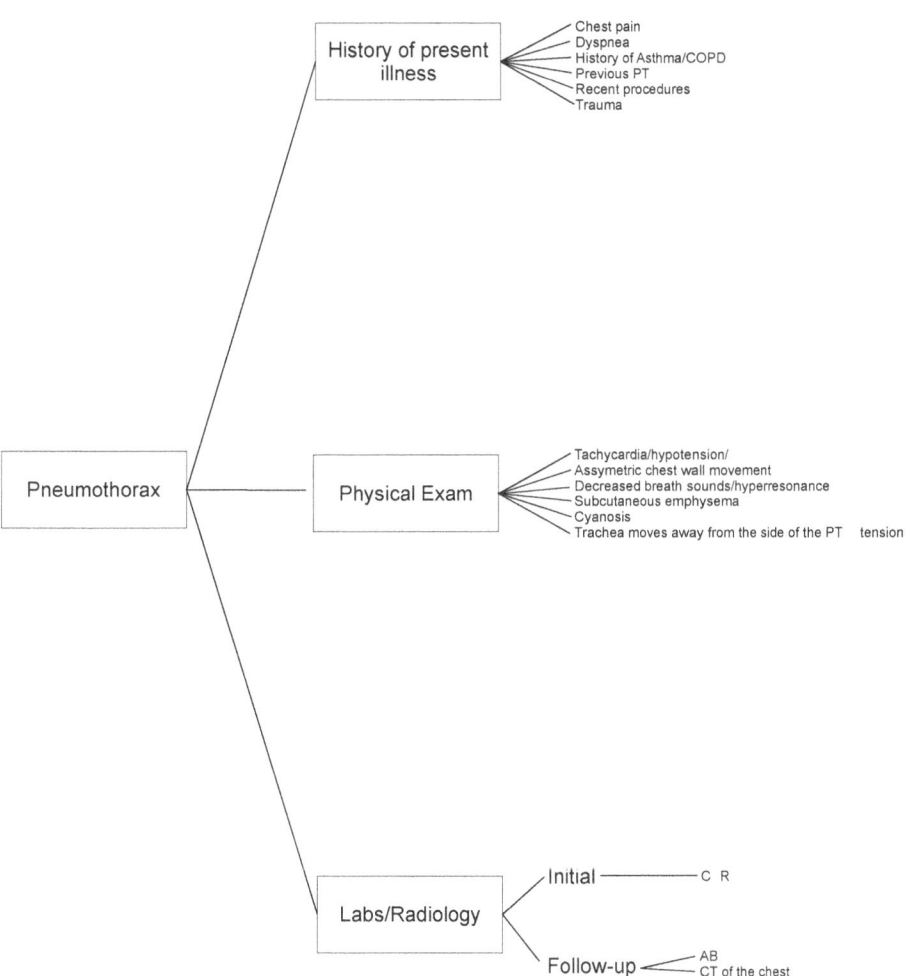

**Pneumothorax**

**History of present illness**
- Chest pain
- Dyspnea
- History of Asthma/COPD
- Previous PT
- Recent procedures
- Trauma

**Physical Exam**
- Tachycardia/hypotension/
- Assymetric chest wall movement
- Decreased breath sounds/hyperresonance
- Subcutaneous emphysema
- Cyanosis
- Trachea moves away from the side of the PT    tension

**Labs/Radiology**
- Initial ——— C R
- Follow-up
  - AB
  - CT of the chest

# Portal Hypertension

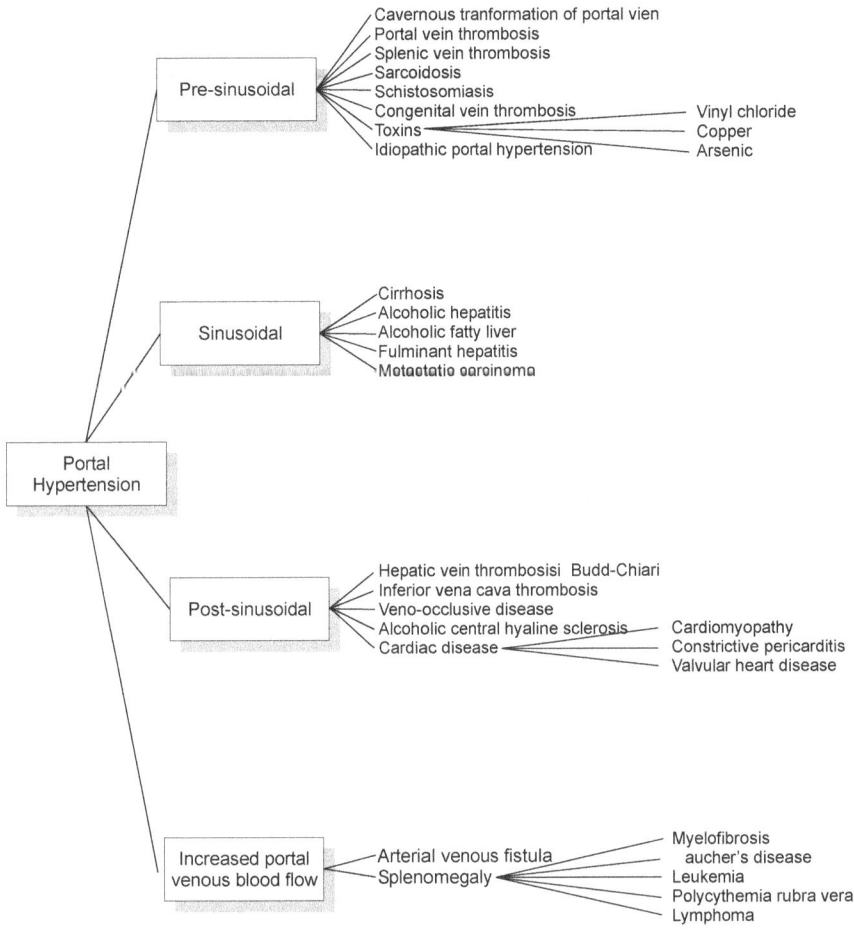

Andreili T, Bennett J, Carpenter C, Plum F, Smith L, Cecil Essentials of Medicine, ed 3, Philadelphia, 1993, W.B. Saunders Company. page 339

# Portal Hypertension

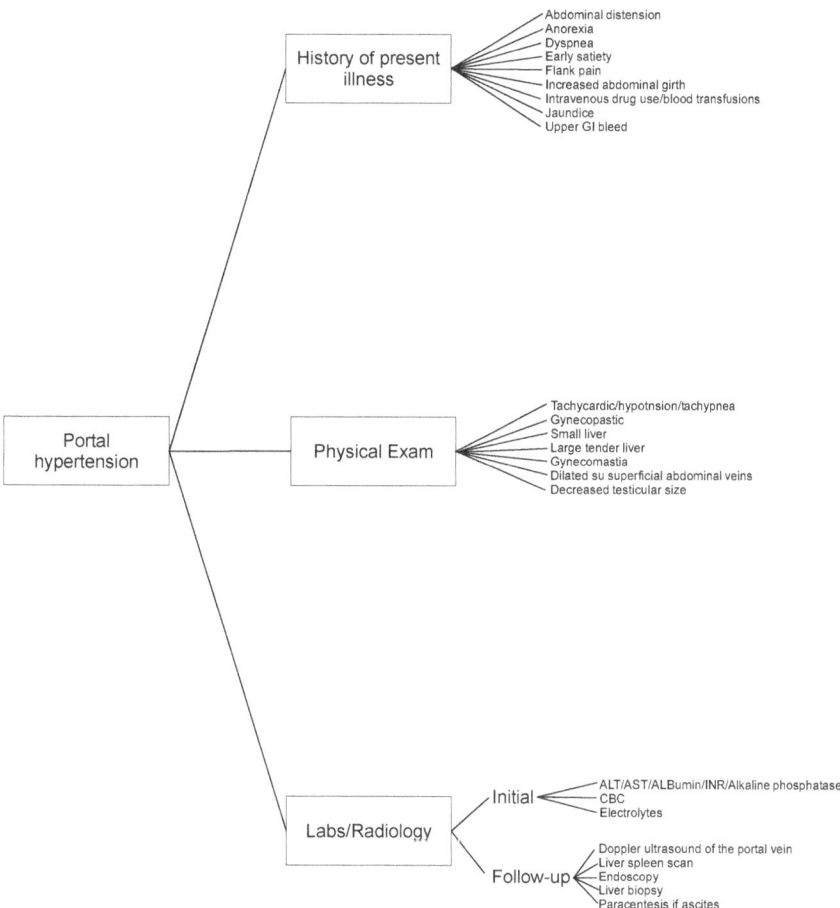

# Pulseless Electrical Activity

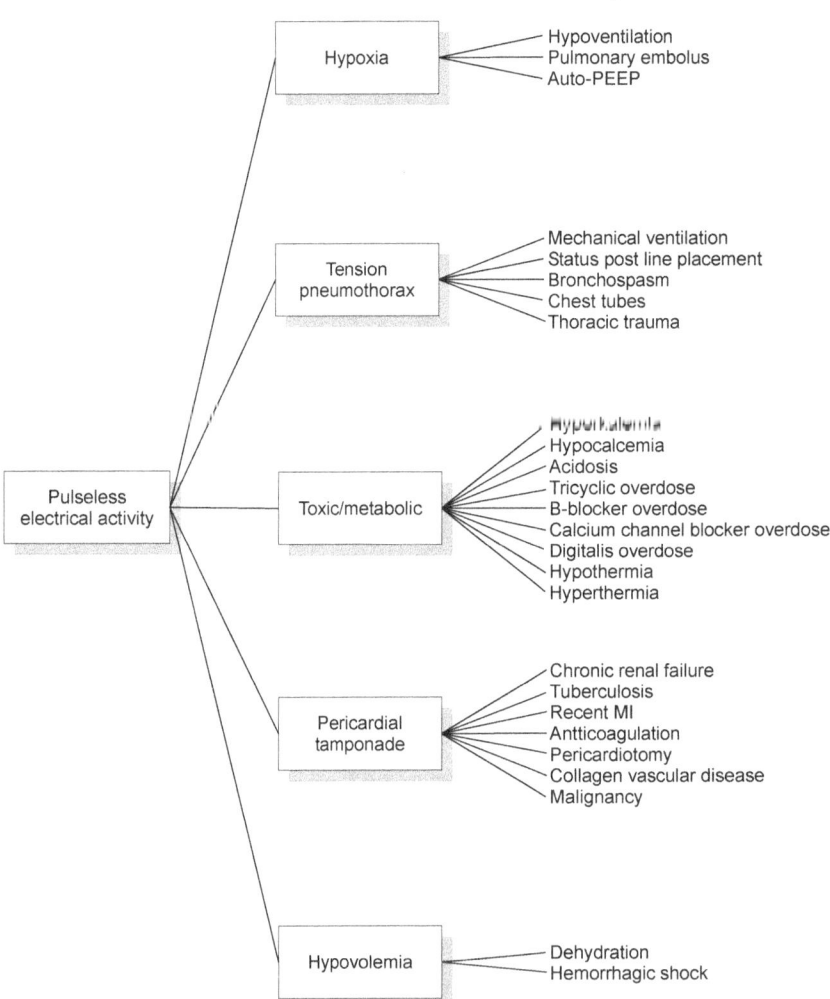

Reference: Slovis C, Wrenn K. The technique of managing pulseless electrical activity. The Journal of Critical Illness 1997;12(11):722-731.

# Acute Renal Failure

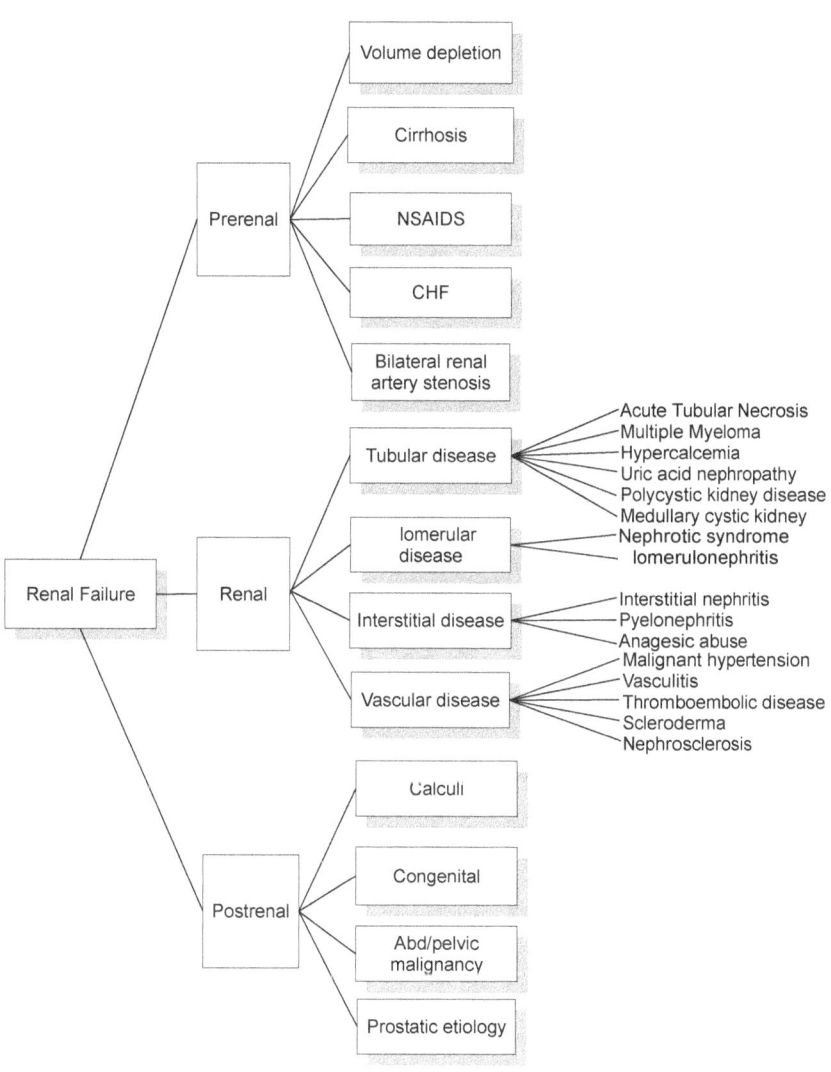

Reference  Kelley, Essentials In Internal Medicine, ed 3  Philadelphia,     4,J B  Lippincott, page 24

# Right Heart Catheterization

| | | | | |
|---|---|---|---|---|
| Normal | Arterial BP | PCWP 4 | CO 2 2 | |
| Hypovolemia | Arterial BP | PCWP 4 | CO 2 2 | Volume expansion |
| Right ventricular infarct | Arterial BP | PCWP 4 | CO 2 2 CVP | Optomize PCWP Dobutamine |
| Pulmonary congestion pulmonary edema | Arterial BP | PCWP | CI 2 2 | Diuretics/Nitroglycerine |
| Low output pulmonary edema | Arterial BP | PCWP | CI 2 2 | Arterial vasodilators |
| Low output pulmonary edema | Arterial BP | PCWP | CI 2 2 | Ionotropic agents Vasodilators Circulatory assistance |
| Mitral regurgitation | Arterial BP variable | PCPW V Wave | CI usually 2 2 | Arterial vasodilators |
| Ventricular septal defect | Arterial BP | PCPW usually | CI variable O2 stepup | Arterial vasodilators |

Reference: Ermakov S, Hoyt J. Pulmonary artery catheterization. Critical Care Clinics 1992;8(4):773-806.

# Seizure

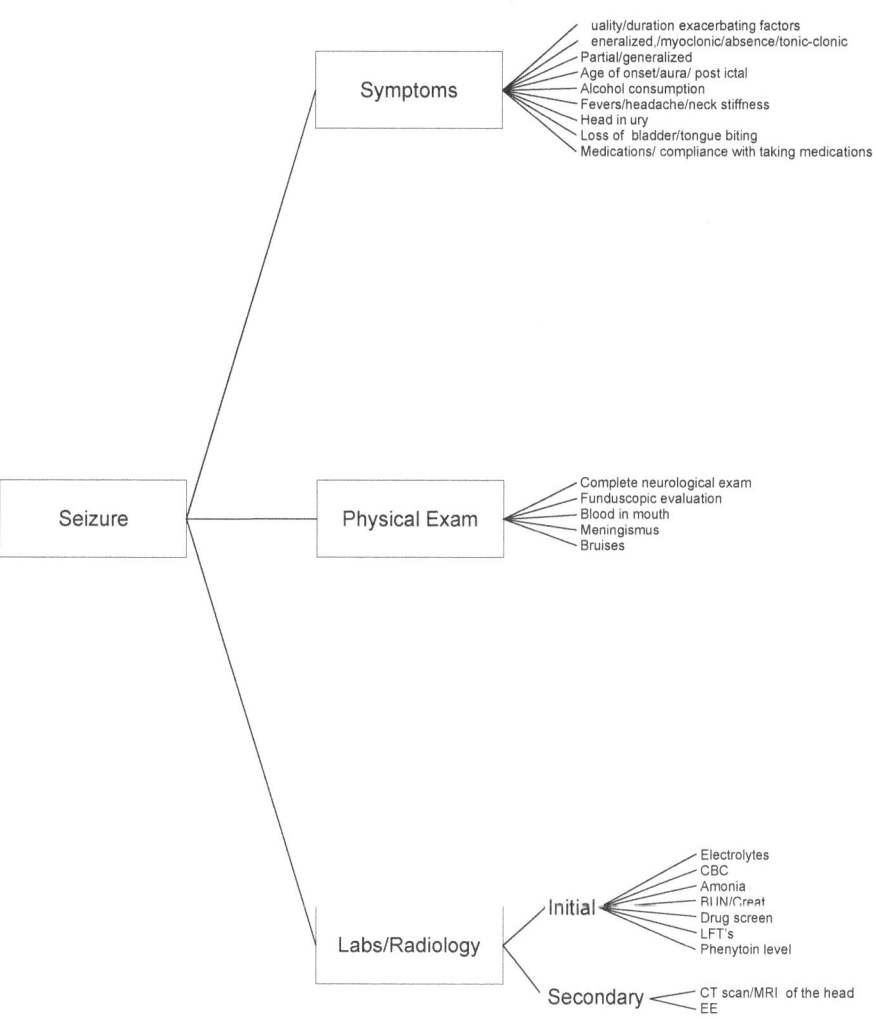

Seizure

**Symptoms**
- uality/duration exacerbating factors
- eneralized,/myoclonic/absence/tonic-clonic
- Partial/generalized
- Age of onset/aura/ post ictal
- Alcohol consumption
- Fevers/headache/neck stiffness
- Head in ury
- Loss of  bladder/tongue biting
- Medications/ compliance with taking medications

**Physical Exam**
- Complete neurological exam
- Funduscopic evaluation
- Blood in mouth
- Meningismus
- Bruises

**Labs/Radiology**

Initial
- Electrolytes
- CBC
- Amonia
- BUN/Creat
- Drug screen
- LFT's
- Phenytoin level

Secondary
- CT scan/MRI  of the head
- EE

# Seizures

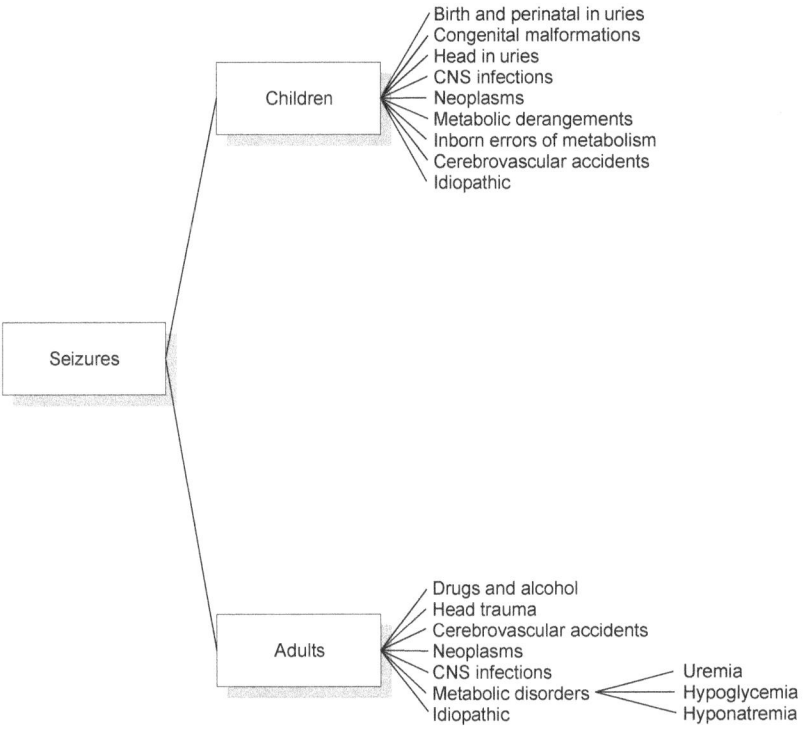

Reference: Sirven J, Liporace J. New antiepileptic drugs. Overcoming the limitations of traditional therapy. Postgraduate Med 1997;102(1):147-50,59-60.

# Shock

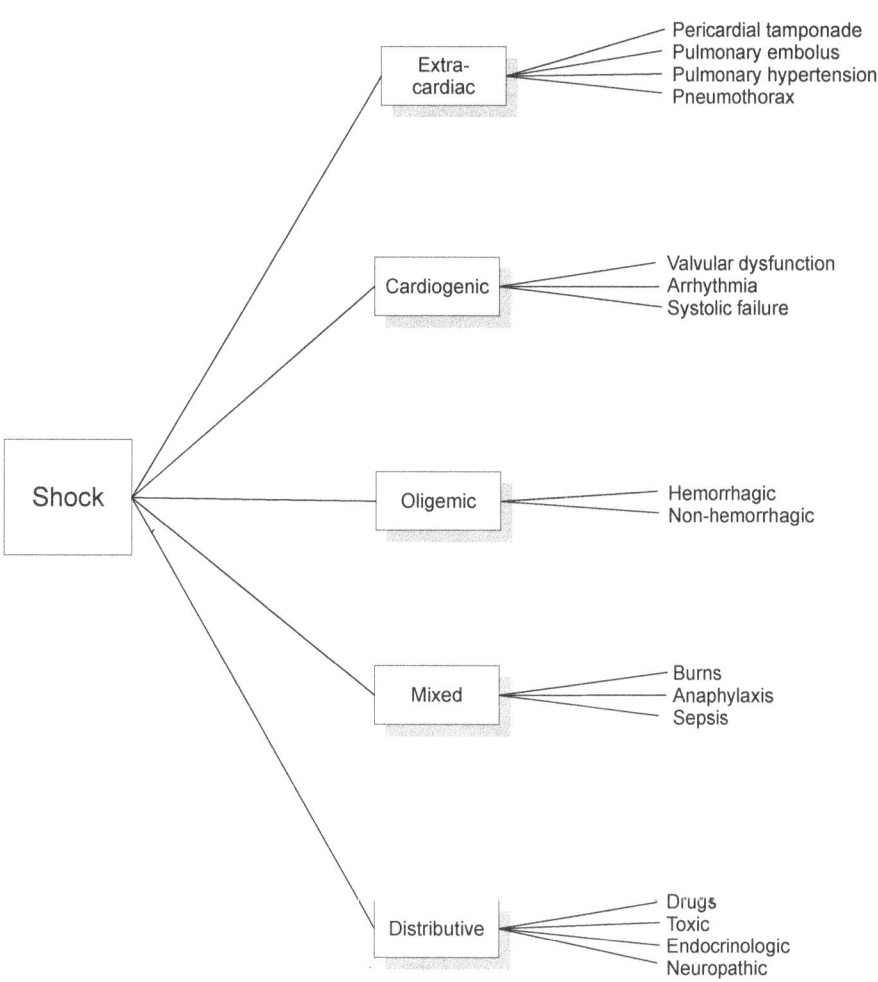

Reference  Parillo J  Pathogenetic mechanisms of septic shock  N Engl J Med    3 32    4   -

# Shock

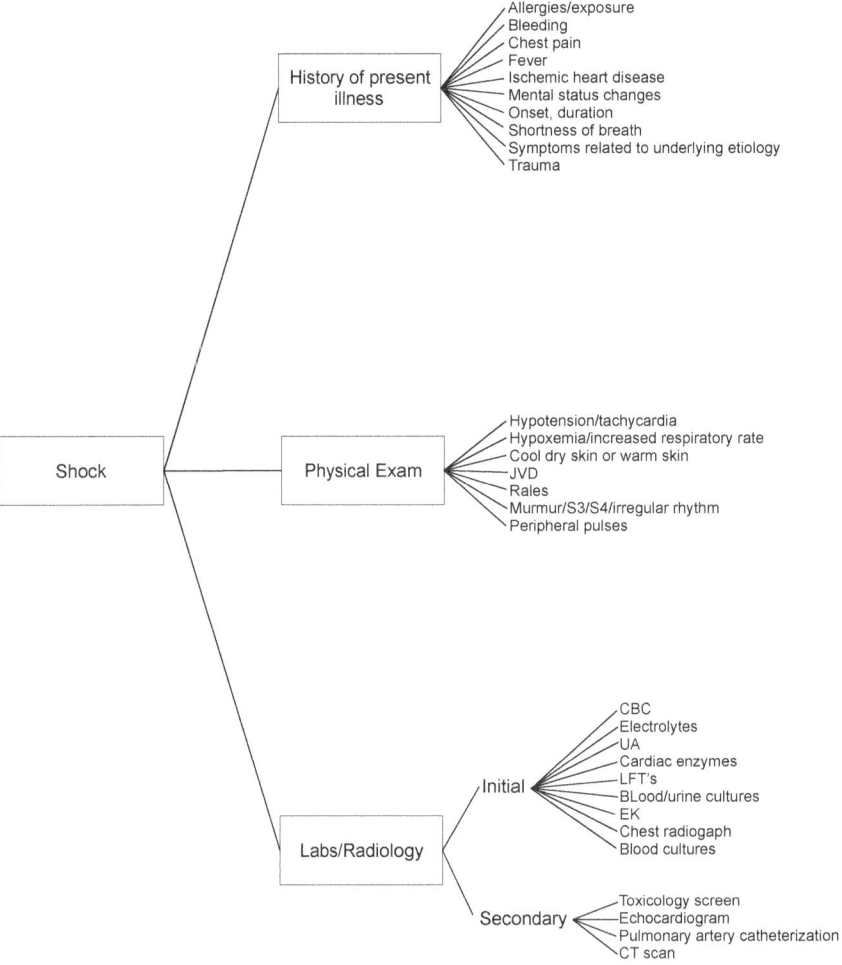

Shock

History of present illness
- Allergies/exposure
- Bleeding
- Chest pain
- Fever
- Ischemic heart disease
- Mental status changes
- Onset, duration
- Shortness of breath
- Symptoms related to underlying etiology
- Trauma

Physical Exam
- Hypotension/tachycardia
- Hypoxemia/increased respiratory rate
- Cool dry skin or warm skin
- JVD
- Rales
- Murmur/S3/S4/irregular rhythm
- Peripheral pulses

Labs/Radiology

Initial
- CBC
- Electrolytes
- UA
- Cardiac enzymes
- LFT's
- BLood/urine cultures
- EK
- Chest radiogaph
- Blood cultures

Secondary
- Toxicology screen
- Echocardiogram
- Pulmonary artery catheterization
- CT scan

# Superior Vena Cava Syndrome

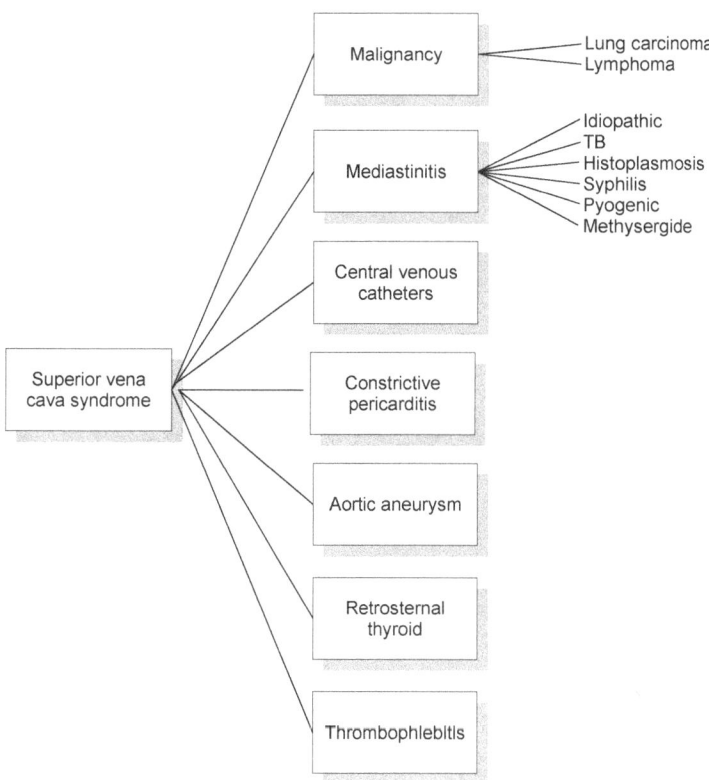

Reference: Markman M. Diagnosis and management of superior vena cava syndrome. Cleve Clin J Med 1999;66(1):59-61

# Superior Vena Cava Syndrome

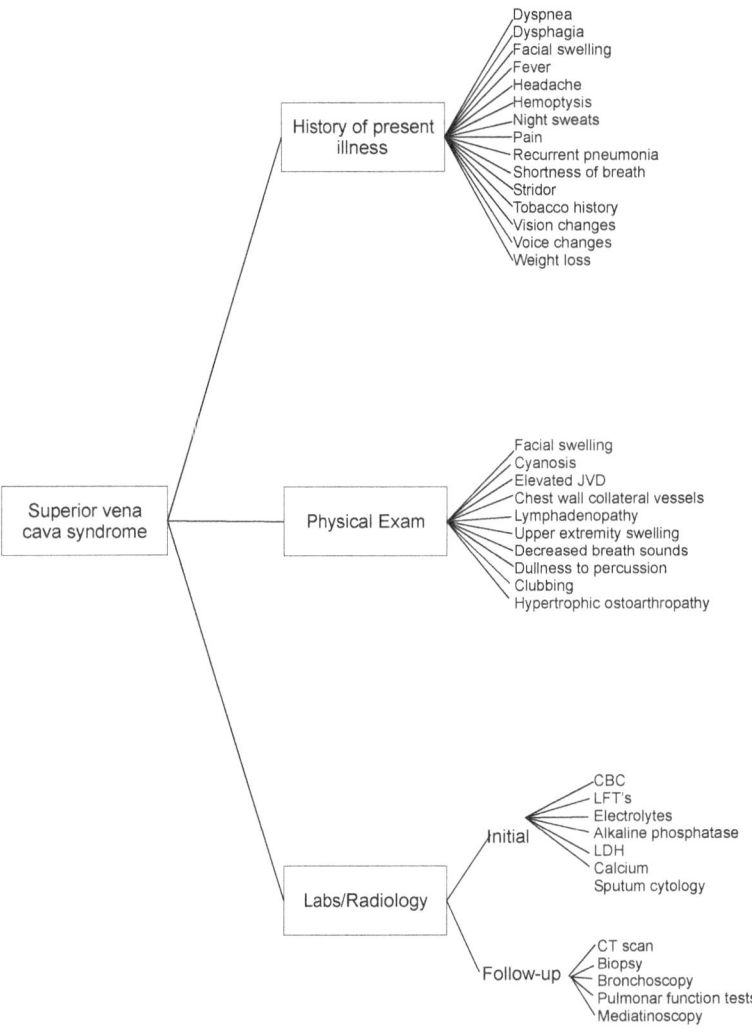

# Ventricular Tachycardia

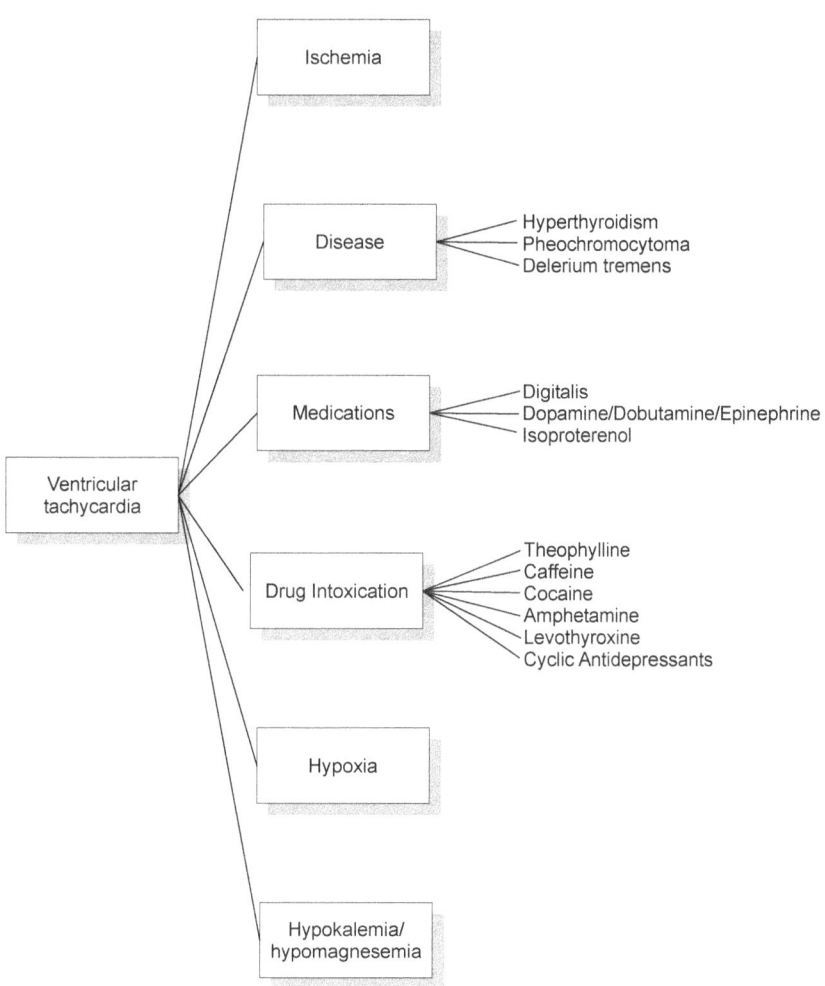

# Ventricular Tachycardia

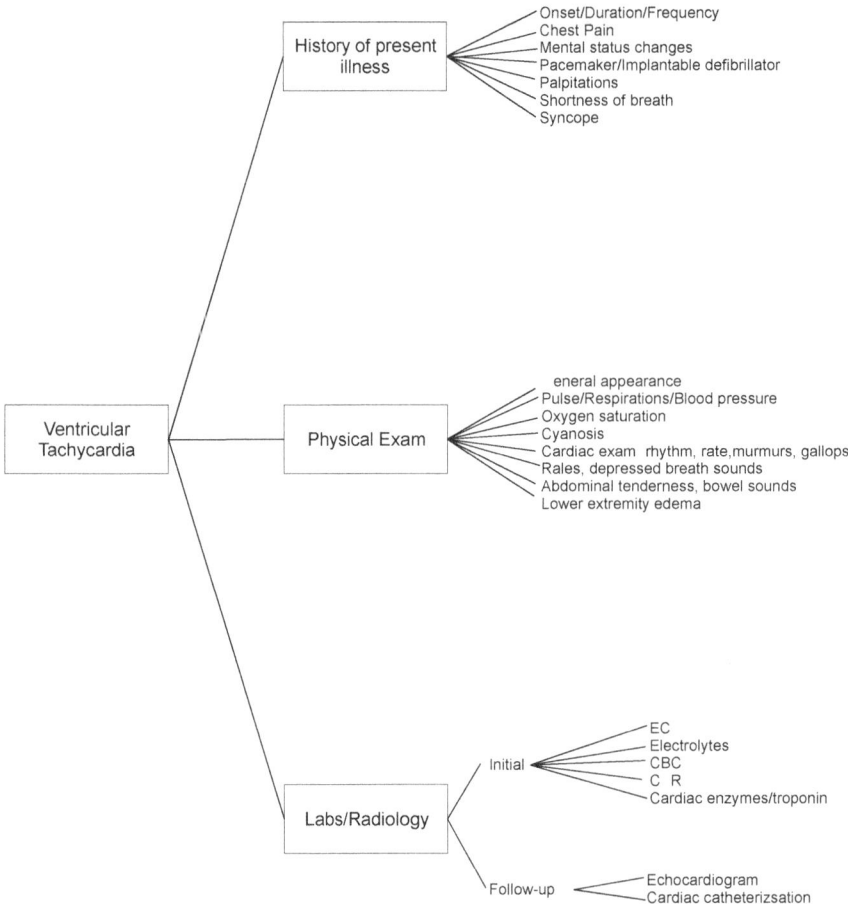

**Ventricular Tachycardia**

**History of present illness**
- Onset/Duration/Frequency
- Chest Pain
- Mental status changes
- Pacemaker/Implantable defibrillator
- Palpitations
- Shortness of breath
- Syncope

**Physical Exam**
- eneral appearance
- Pulse/Respirations/Blood pressure
- Oxygen saturation
- Cyanosis
- Cardiac exam  rhythm, rate,murmurs, gallops
- Rales, depressed breath sounds
- Abdominal tenderness, bowel sounds
- Lower extremity edema

**Labs/Radiology**

Initial
- EC
- Electrolytes
- CBC
- C  R
- Cardiac enzymes/troponin

Follow-up
- Echocardiogram
- Cardiac catheterizsation

This concludes Differential Diagnosis Diagrams:

Fast Focus Study Guide

Search Amazon or other book retailers to find other books in the

Fast Focus Study Guide Series

Search Amazon Print Books and Kindle books to find other study guides written by

JT Thomas, MD

Internal Medicine Study Guide

Hematology Study Guide

Medical Oncology Study Guide

Cardiology Study Guide

Nephrology Study Guide

Multiple Myeloma Study Guide

Differential Diagnosis Study Guide

Ovarian Cancer Study Guide

Rheumatology Study Guide

Cancer Study Guide

www.ingramcontent.com/pod-product-compliance
Lightning Source LLC
Chambersburg PA
CBHW080818180526
45168CB00006B/2495